Understanding

ELECTROCARDIOGRAPHY

Physiological and interpretive concepts

MARY BOUDREAU CONOVER, R.N., B.S.N.Ed.

Consulting Instructor in Critical Care,
Basic and Advanced Arrhythmia Workshops,
West Hills and West Park Hospitals, Canoga Park, California;
Faculty, National Critical Care Institute, Orange, California

Contributor

EDWARD L. CONOVER, B.S.E.E.

THIRD EDITION

*With **411** illustrations*

The C. V. Mosby Company

ST. LOUIS • TORONTO • LONDON   1980

THIRD EDITION

Copyright © 1980 by The C. V. Mosby Company

All rights reserved. No part of this book may be reproduced
in any manner without written permission of the publisher.

Previous editions copyrighted 1972 and 1976

Printed in the United States of America

The C. V. Mosby Company
11830 Westline Industrial Drive, St. Louis, Missouri 63141

Library of Congress Cataloging in Publication Data

Conover, Mary Boudreau, 1931-
　　Understanding electrocardiography.

　　Bibliography: p.
　　Includes index.
　　1.　Electrocardiography.　I.　Title.　[DNLM:
1.　Electrocardiography.　WG140 C753u]
RC683.5.E5C65　1980　　　616.1'207547　　　80-14104
ISBN　0-8016-5676-1

GW/VH/VH　9　8　7　6　5　4　3　2　1　　　03/D/341

Understanding

ELECTROCARDIOGRAPHY

Physiological and interpretive concepts

Lovingly dedicated to
my husband
Edward

Consulting board

S. SERGE BAROLD, M.B., F.R.A.C.P., F.A.C.P., F.A.C.C.

Chief of Cardiology, The Genesee Hospital; Associate Professor of Medicine,
University of Rochester School of Medicine and Dentistry, Rochester,
New York

HENRY J. L. MARRIOTT, M.D., F.A.C.P., F.A.C.C.

Director of Clinical Research, Rogers Heart Foundation; Director of
Coronary Care Center and Director of Electrocardiograph Department,
St. Anthony's Hospital, St. Petersburg, Florida; Clinical Professor
of Medicine (Cardiology), Emory University School of Medicine,
Atlanta, Georgia; Clinical Professor of Pediatrics (Cardiology),
University of Florida, Gainesville, Florida

MICHAEL ROSEN, M.D.

Associate Professor, Department of Pharmacology and Pediatrics,
College of Physicians and Surgeons, Columbia University,
New York, New York

HEIN J. J. WELLENS, M.D.

Professor of Medicine and Chief of Cardiology, University of Limburg,
Maastricht, The Netherlands

Preface

Rapid, accurate arrhythmia detection and identification involve an understanding of electrocardiography solidly based on anatomy, physiology, electrophysiology, and arrhythmogenesis. This book, intended for both the beginner and the advanced student of electrocardiography, presents such information, with emphasis on mechanism and causes, in the firm belief that the approach facilitates a correct diagnosis. Chapters 1 through 9 are especially suited for a course in basic electrocardiography, whereas Chapters 10 through 19 are more easily assimilated after the basics are well in hand.

In this third edition of *Understanding Electrocardiography* almost every chapter has been completely rewritten in light of the most recent information available on the mechanisms and causes of arrhythmias. Following is a summary of the most pertinent changes and additions:

1. Wolff-Parkinson-White syndrome is taking on more and more significance as a cause of paroxysmal supraventricular tachycardia, atrial fibrillation, and primary ventricular fibrillation. Many of the important studies regarding this syndrome have been carried out by Dr. Hein J. J. Wellens of The Netherlands. I am indebted to him for reviewing this chapter and supplying me with his most recent research paper for my main reference.

2. The material on supraventricular ectopics has been reorganized and reclassified: the result has been to clarify terminology and better define an approach to treatment. An important addition to this chapter is the correct monitoring procedure in acute myocardial infarction. Dr. Henry J. L. Marriott reviewed this chapter, as well as those on bundle branch block, hemiblock, and aberrant ventricular conduction. I am grateful to him for this and for his encouragement.

3. The chapters on electrophysiology and arrhythmogenesis were reviewed by Dr. Michael Rosen who advised me on the important addition of afterpotentials as a cause of arrhythmias.

4. The chapter on pacemakers has been totally rewritten and includes methods for evaluating the functions of the demand pacemaker, as well as the more common causes and manifestations of pacemaker

malfunction. I am grateful to Dr. S. Serge Barold for reviewing this chapter.

5. Any chapter on pacemakers is incomplete without a discussion of accidental electrocution of the electrically sensitive patient. This important chapter has been thoroughly researched and brought up to date by the original contributor, Edward L. Conover, B.S.E.E. I am most appreciative of this contribution by an expert in the field.

6. The chapter on myocardial infarction has been extensively revised, especially the section dealing with the electrophysiology of the normal S-T segment and S-T segment elevation, which was reviewed by Dr. Borys Surawicz. I am indebted to him. In addition, many new 12-lead electrocardiograms have been added to better illustrate how to determine the area of infarction.

7. The chapter on drugs has been completely rewritten to include new antiarrhythmics and new information on antiarrhythmics of long standing. I would like to express my gratitude to Dr. Ara G. Tilkian for reviewing this chapter for me.

8. Chapter 20 is a collection of test tracings, originally found at the end of each chapter, and is offered for self-evaluation and for experience in arrhythmia detection.

9. An often-requested glossary has been added at the end of the book. Because research in electrophysiology and the mechanisms of arrhythmias has moved so rapidly in the last ten years, terms evolve that cannot be found in the standard medical dictionary simply because they are too new for standard usage.

Dr. Leonard Lyon, who was kind enough to read the second edition, made specific suggestions for the third. I would like to take this opportunity to thank him.

The new illustrations in this and previous editions were expertly drawn by René Fontan.

Finally, as in the past, I am grateful to the CCU nurses of West Park Hospital, Canoga Park, California, who so faithfully collected rhythm strips and 12-lead electrocardiograms for me.

Mary Boudreau Conover

Contents

CHAPTER 1

Anatomy and physiology of the heart

The heart as a pump

The four chambers of the heart function as a double pump. The right side of the heart propels venous blood to the lungs for oxygenation, while the left side of the heart propels oxygenated blood into the systemic circulation.

During diastole both atria and ventricles are filling with blood. Atrial systole adds the last complement of blood to the ventricles (end-diastolic pressure) before they contract.

Venous blood enters the right atrium by way of the superior and the inferior vena cava, while oxygenated blood enters the left atrium by way of the four pulmonary veins. There are no valves separating these vessels from the atrial chambers.

The tricuspid valve separates the right atrium from the right ventricle, while the mitral valve separates the left atrium from the left ventricle. When ventricular systole commences, these valves close to prevent a reflux of blood into the atrial chambers.

Ventricular systole propels the blood through the semilunar valves into the pulmonary artery and the aorta. When diastole begins, the aortic and pulmonic valves close so that a return of blood to the ventricles is prevented.

The flow of blood through the heart's chambers, vessels, and valves is illustrated in Fig. 1-1.

Papillary muscles and the chordae tendineae

The atrioventricular (AV) valves (mitral and tricuspid) are prevented from bulging back into the atria during ventricular systole by slender, strong cords (chordae tendineae). These cords extend from the borders of the valves to fingerlike projections on the ventricular walls (papillary muscles). When the ventricles contract, so do the papillary muscles, causing the chordae tendineae to restrain the valve leaflets from inverting into the atria.

Fig. 1-1 illustrates the chordae tendineae and papillary muscles of the heart. Note that the left ventricle has two papillary muscles with chordae tendineae to the two cusps of the mitral valve. In the right ventricle there are usually three papillary muscles with chordae tendineae to the three cusps of the tricuspid valve.

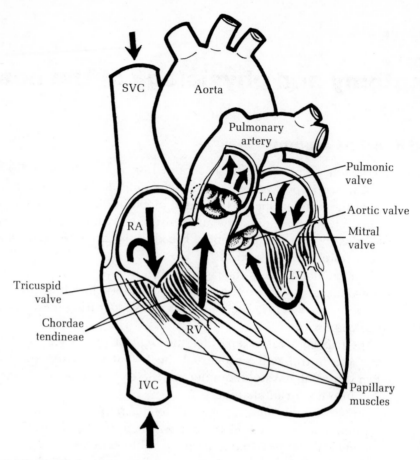

Fig. 1-1. Course of the blood through the chambers, valves, and vessels of the heart. *SVC,* Superior vena cava; *IVC,* inferior vena cava. The papillary muscles and chordae tendineae are also shown. (From Tilkian, A. G., and Conover, M. H.: Understanding heart sounds and murmurs, Philadelphia, 1979, W. B. Saunders Co.)

Surfaces of the heart

The heart has four surfaces: anterior, posterior, diaphragmatic, and lateral (Fig. 1-2). The anterior and posterior surfaces oppose each other on one plane; the lateral and diaphragmatic surfaces oppose each other on another plane.

Conductive system of the heart

Before the heart can contract, it must be stimulated to do so, the stimulus being delivered quickly and efficiently to all areas of the myocardium. These two functions—self-excitation and rapid conduction velocity—are ac-

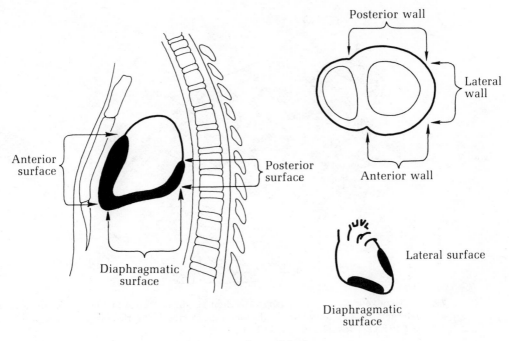

Fig. 1-2. Surfaces of the heart.

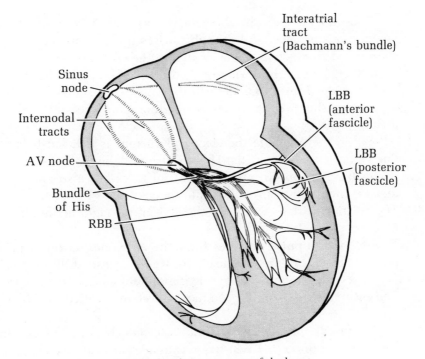

Fig. 1-3. Conductive system of the heart.

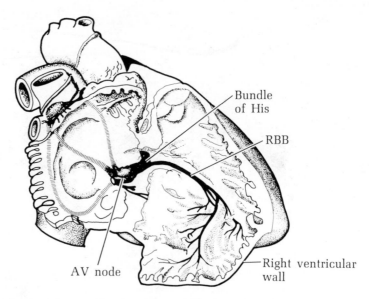

Bundle
of His

RBB

AV node

Right ventricular
wall

Fig. 1-4. Right ventricle opened to show the right bundle branch with its branches to the septum and to the anterior papillary muscle. (From Marriott, H. J. L.: Workshop in electrocardiography, Tampa Tracings, Oldsmar, Fla., 1972.)

complished by a specialized conductive system. Automatically and at regular intervals an electrical stimulus arises in the sinus node, a grouping of specialized conductive tissue located in the right atrium adjacent to the superior vena cava. The atria are then depolarized, and the impulse invades the AV node. James[1] has described tracts of specialized conductive tissue connecting the two nodes and extending from the sinus node to the left atrium.

Within the AV node the electrical current is delayed before being conducted to the bundle of His. This consistent delay not only protects the ventricles from inappropriately high atrial rates but also allows time for the atrial contents to be propelled into the ventricles before the latter contract. The position of the AV node in the floor of the right atrium is illustrated in Figs. 1-3 and 1-4.

After the impulse emerges from the AV node, its rapid propagation is resumed by way of the bundle of His. Rapid spread of the current within the ventricles is accomplished by the bundle branches and their ramifications. The entire interventricular conductive system is called the His-Purkinje system.

The bundle of His divides into two main branches, right and left. The right bundle branch (RBB) has terminal ramifications in the lower interventricular (IV) septum and the wall of the right ventricle. This is diagram-

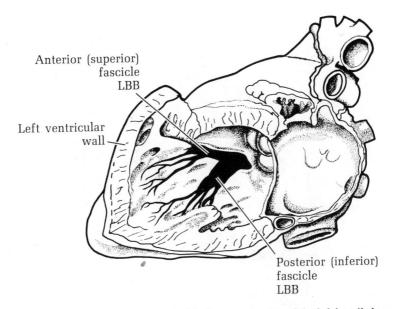

Anterior (superior)
fascicle
LBB

Left ventricular
wall

Posterior (inferior)
fascicle
LBB

Fig. 1-5. Left ventricle opened to show a simplified representation of the left bundle branch with its anterior (superior) and posterior (inferior) divisions. (From Marriott, H. J. L.: Workshop in electrocardiography, Tampa Tracings, Oldsmar, Fla., 1972.)

matically illustrated in Figs. 1-3 and 1-4. The left bundle branch (LBB) is thought by some authorities to have two distinct fascicles, one to the anterior wall and one to the posterior wall of the left ventricle. Others believe that this is an oversimplification. However, the concept of two distinct fascicles is useful in the understanding of hemiblock. The LBB and its ramifications are simplified and diagrammatically illustrated in Figs. 1-3 and 1-5. Fig. 1-5 views the left ventricle from the side, showing that the anterior fascicle is superior and the posterior fascicle inferior.

Atrioventricular (AV) junction

A ring of fibrous tissue surrounds each of the four valves of the heart. This fibrous skeleton will not conduct electrical current. Normally the sole muscular connection between the upper and lower chambers of the heart is that part of the specialized conductive system known as the bundle of His. The AV node and the nonbranching portion of the bundle of His are called the AV junction. Normal ventricular activation depends on an intact and healthy pathway across this junction. Fig. 1-6 is a highly magnified diagrammatic representation of the AV junction. The depolarization wave front is shown entering the AV node, traversing it, and arriving at the bundle of His in a uniform wave front.

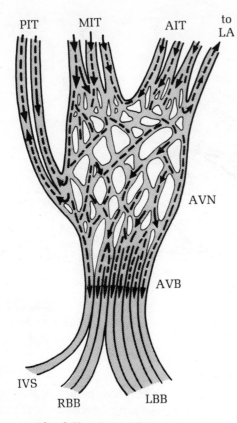

Fig. 1-6. The AV junction. *PIT*, Posterior internodal tract; *MIT*, middle internodal tract; *AIT*, anterior internodal tract; *LA*, left atrium; *AVN*, AV node; *AVB*, His (AV) bundle; *IVS*, direct connections to the interventricular septum; *RBB* and *LBB*, right and left bundle branches. Black arrows indicate the direction of spread of excitation. Many authorities believe that the existence of well-defined specific internodal pathways is not a proven anatomical fact. (From Sherf, L., and James, T. N.: Am. J. Cardiol. **29:** 529, 1972.)

The following abbreviations are commonly used to refer to specific parts of the AV junction: AN (atrionodal), where the internodal tracts become nodal tissue; N (nodal), specifically nodal tissue; and NH (nodal-His), where the nodal tissue becomes the bundle of His. (The N region is said to be the only part of the conductive system not possessing pacemaker cells.)

Properties of cardiac muscle

There are three types of cardiac muscle: atrial, ventricular, and noncontractile muscle fibers of the conductive system. These muscles have four primary characteristics: excitability, automaticity, conductivity, and contractility.

EXCITABILITY

Excitability refers to the ability of the cell to reach threshold in response to a stimulus. The smaller the stimulus requirement, the higher the excitability, and vice versa.

The cardiac muscle is electrically irritable because of an ionic imbalance

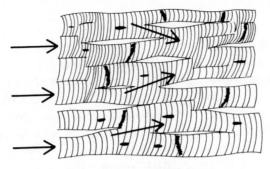

Fig. 1-7. Electrical current spreading along the axis and laterally through the unique interconnections of cardiac muscle.

across the membranes of the cells. The degree of negativity within the cell determines its excitability, or *responsiveness*.

AUTOMATICITY

Automaticity is that property by which a cell can reach a threshold potential and generate an action potential without being stimulated from another source.

In pacemaker cells there is a regular, cyclic fall in potassium conduction during diastole. This, along with an increased permeability to sodium, causes a threshold to be reached and an action potential to occur at regular intervals. Thus a current is initiated and propagated along the membranes of all the myocardial cells. This property of cardiac pacemaker cells will be discussed in more detail in Chapter 2.

CONDUCTIVITY

Conductivity refers to the propagation of an impulse from cell to cell.

Conduction velocity is enhanced primarily by the conductive system of the heart that speeds the impulse along at a rate which is six times faster than would be otherwise possible.

The anatomical structure of the heart also influences conduction velocity. Because of a unique interconnection of muscle fibers, the stimulation of a cardiac cell under normal conditions by an impulse that exceeds its threshold potential produces a propagated response.

Fig. 1-7 is a representation of the many lateral and end-to-side connections in cardiac muscle. The electrical current spreads from cell to cell along the axis and laterally through the interconnections more rapidly than in skeletal muscle.

Conduction velocity is also dependent on cellular physiology, which is discussed in Chapter 2.

CONTRACTILITY

The contractility of cardiac muscle refers to the ability of the fibers to shorten when stimulated, a property dependent on many factors. Normally the myocardium contracts in response to electrical current generated in the sinus node and propagated through the entire heart.

An increase in myocardial contractility occurs with digitalis, bretylium, sympathomimetics, hypercalcemia, and hyperthyroidism. Increased contractility as a compensatory mechanism occurs in response to increased venous return to the heart, exercise, emotion, hypovolemia, and anemia.

A decrease in myocardial contractility occurs with quinidine, procainamide, beta blocking agents, hyperkalemia, hypocalcemia, hypothyroidism, shock, and diffuse myocardial disease.

Conduction time through the heart: the His bundle electrogram (HBE)

The standard electrocardiogram (ECG) records only the atrial and ventricular electrical events. The actual firing of the sinus node and conduction of the impulse across the AV junction are not represented. The latter can be inferred from the relationship of the atrial wave to the ventricular complex. Exact time values can be obtained for the progress of the current through the AV junction by positioning a bipolar recording catheter at the tricuspid valve. (See p. 2.) This record is known as the His bundle electrogram. At the same time, an atrial electrogram (A) and ventricular electrogram (V) are also obtained.

With the His bundle electrogram conduction can be separated into two main divisions: (1) from the onset of the P wave to the activation of the bundle of His, called the PH interval, and (2) from His bundle activation to the onset of the QRS complex (ventricular activation), known as the HR interval. These measurements are shown in Fig. 1-8. Other measurements are PA, extending from the onset of the P wave to the onset of the atrial electrogram, and AH, from the atrial component to the His bundle component.

Sinus, or sinoatrial (SA), node as pacemaker of the heart

Because the sinus node cycles more rapidly than any other part of the conductive system, it paces the heart. Under abnormal conditions other areas of the heart may usurp this control, by more rapid cycling or by passively taking over, either because the normal pacemaker has failed or because it is generating its impulses too slowly.

The pacemaker cells have an intrinsic rate that becomes slower and slower from the sinus node down to the end of the His-Purkinje system. The

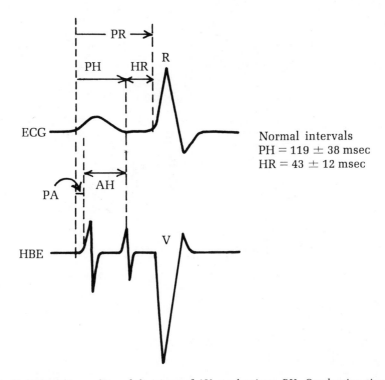

Normal intervals
PH = 119 ± 38 msec
HR = 43 ± 12 msec

Fig. 1-8. Electrocardiographic subdivisions of AV conductions. *PH*, Conduction time through atria, AV node, and His bundle; *HR*, time from the onset of the His deflection to the onset of ventricular deflection. (From Hecht, H. H., et al.: Am. J. Cardiol. **31:**232, 1973.)

AV node itself is thought to have no pacemaker cells and hence no power of automaticity. Its chief function is to delay the impulse in order to allow for adequate ventricular filling. However, the bundle of His has pacemaker cells that are capable of discharging at a rhythmic rate of 40 to 60 times/min.

Below the bundle of His its branches to their terminal ramifications discharge at a rate of 15 to 40 times/min. Normally the sinus node discharges the other potential pacemakers before self-excitation can occur in them. The sinus node is therefore the pacemaker of the heart. This electrophysiological mechanism is discussed in Chapter 2.

Autonomic nervous system and control of the heart

The autonomic nervous system controls the visceral functions of the body. It distributes impulses to the heart, smooth muscle, and glands. The two divisions of the autonomic nervous system are the sympathetic and parasympathetic systems (Fig. 1-9). A more complete discussion and terminology may be found on pp. 220 to 226.

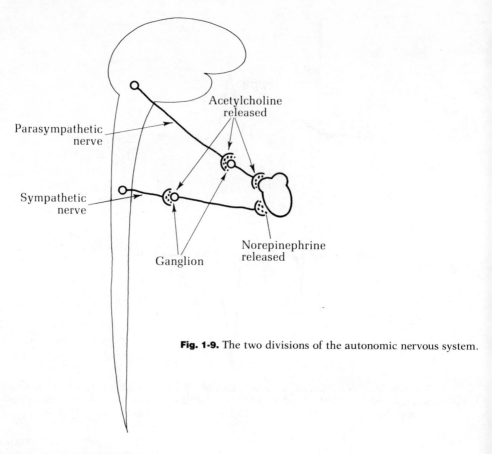

Fig. 1-9. The two divisions of the autonomic nervous system.

SYMPATHETIC NERVES

The sympathetic nerves originate in the spinal cord between the first thoracic and second lumbar vertebrae (T-1 and L-2). They supply both the atria and the ventricles, but chiefly the ventricles. Norepinephrine is the mediator, having the effects of increasing the force of cardiac contraction and enhancing the excitability of the heart. It exerts a moderate effect on the atria by increasing the rate of the sinus node.

PARASYMPATHETIC NERVES

The parasympathetic nerves leave the central nervous system through the cranial and sacral spinal nerves. The vagi are the parasympathetic nerves of the heart (primarily of the atria). Stimulation of the vagi causes the hormone acetylcholine to be released. The effects are mainly supraventricular, causing a slowing in the rate of the sinus node and a decrease in the rate of conduction through the AV node. The ventricles may also receive parasympathetic innervation, probably exclusively to the Purkinje network.[2-6]

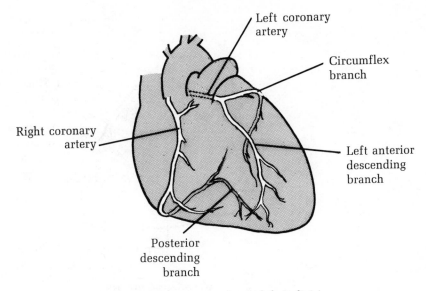

Left coronary artery

Circumflex branch

Right coronary artery

Left anterior descending branch

Posterior descending branch

Fig. 1-10. Coronary arteries and their divisions.

Coronary circulation
CORONARY ARTERIES

As the aorta leaves the heart to supply the tissues of the body with blood, its first debt is paid to the heart muscle itself. The right and left coronary arteries (Fig. 1-10) arise from within the sinuses of Valsalva.

The *right coronary artery* descends from its origin in the aorta and courses along the AV groove (sulcus). It gives off branches to the sinus node in 55% of hearts and to the right atrium and ventricle. It then turns posteriorly around the inferior margin of the heart, sending branches to the AV node in 90% of hearts, as well as to the bundle of His, and to the posterior division of the left bundle branch. The *posterior descending branch* of the right coronary artery supplies nearly half the diaphragmatic (inferior) surface of the left ventricle.

The *left coronary artery* descends from its origin in the aorta to divide into the *circumflex* and *anterior descending branches*. The circumflex branch courses along in the AV groove and turns posteriorly. It supplies the lateral wall of the left ventricle, half the diaphragmatic surface of the left ventricle, the AV node in 10% of hearts, and the sinus node in 45%. The *anterior descending branch* supplies all the bundle branches, the anterior wall of the left ventricle, and part of the right ventricle, as well as the anterior two thirds of the IV septum.

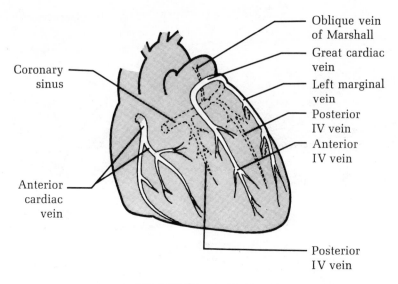

Fig. 1-11. Coronary veins.

CORONARY VEINS

The left ventricle is drained by the largest system of coronary veins—the coronary sinus and its tributaries. In Fig. 1-11 these tributaries can be seen over the left ventricular walls anteriorly, laterally, and posteriorly. In the IV sulcus the *anterior interventricular vein* lies parallel to the anterior descending branch of the left coronary artery. Blood flow in the two vessels is, of course, in opposite directions. At the place where the main left coronary artery usually divides, the anterior IV vein turns toward the left margin of the heart and becomes known as the *great cardiac vein.* Emptying into this vein are the *left marginal* and *posterior interventricular veins.* Posteriorly the great cardiac vein becomes the *coronary sinus* and empties into the right atrium. The *posterior interventricular vein* and the smaller *oblique vein of Marshall* empty into the coronary sinus.

The right ventricle is drained by the *anterior cardiac veins.* These can be seen (Fig. 1-11) over the anterior wall of the right ventricle as two or three large trunks draining toward the right AV sulcus to empty into the right atrium.

The smallest system of veins is known as the *Thebesian veins.* These small veins occur primarily in the right atrium and right ventricle and drain directly into the cardiac chambers.

Summary

The heart is a double pump in which both halves share the same conductive system, which is composed of the sinoatrial (SA), or sinus node, internodal and interatrial tracts, the AV node, bundle of His, and bundle branches. All the structures of the conductive system except the AV node possess the property of self-excitation, whereas atrial and ventricular muscle does not. The sinus node paces the heart because it cycles more rapidly than do the other pacemaker cells.

The heart is under the control of the autonomic nervous system and receives its blood supply from the right and left coronary arteries and their branches. The right coronary artery supplies the AV node and the inferior wall of the left ventricle. The left coronary artery mainly supplies all the bundle branches, the left ventricle, and the IV septum.

References

1. James, T. N.: The connecting pathways between the sinus node and AV node and between the right and left atriums in the human heart, Am. Heart J. **66:**498, 1963.
2. Lyon, L. J., and Nevins, M. A.: Retching and termination of ventricular tachycardia, Chest **74:**110, 1978.
3. Scherf, D., Cohen, J., and Raflzadeh, M.: Excitatory effects of carotid sinus pressure, Am. J. Cardiol. **17:**240, 1966.
4. Waxman, M. B., and Wald, R. W.: Termination of ventricular tachycardia by an increase in cardiac vagal drive, Circulation **56:**385, 1977.
5. Weiss, T., Lattin, G. M., and Engleman, K.: Vagally mediated suppression of premature ventricular contractions in man, Am. Heart J. **89:**700, 1975.
6. Kent, K. K., Smith, E. R., Redwood, D. R., and Epstein, S. E.: Electrical stability of acutely ischemic myocardium. Influence of heart rate and vagal stimulation, Circulation **47:**291, 1973.

CHAPTER 2

Electrophysiology of the normal heart

Current flow in the heart

The physiological events that precede the mechanical acts of contraction and relaxation are electrochemical in nature. The fluids both inside and outside the cell membranes of the body are electrolyte solutions made up of negative and positive ions. Current will flow between ions of opposite polarity if they are together within a suitable conductive medium. The current flows from the negative ions to the positive ions in the extracellular fluid.

When the muscle cells of the heart are at rest, the intracellular fluid is mostly negative. Thus there will be no current flow between cells. But when a muscle cell of the heart is stimulated, there is a change in polarity across the membrane of the cell. Its interior becomes positively charged due to the entry of positively charged sodium (Na^+) ions. A difference then exists between this cell and its neighbor, and a current discharges, or flows, between the two until all cells in the same muscle mass have been stimulated to change their polarity.

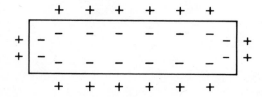

Fig. 2-1. Resting cell.

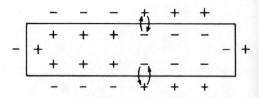

Fig. 2-2. Depolarization.

Resting membrane potential

In between electrical impulses the cell is said to be at rest. The electrical potential existing across the cell membrane during this time is called the *resting membrane potential,* which consists of an accumulation of negative ions along the inner surface of the cell membrane and an equal accumulation of positive ions on the outer surface of the membrane. Fig. 2-1 is a diagrammatic illustration of the resting cell, which is said to be *polarized.*

An electrode inserted across the membrane into the inside of the cell records a difference in potential between the inside and the outside of the cell of −90 millivolts (mV). This electrical potential exists across the membrane of healthy cells in the atria and ventricles. Any decline of this membrane potential to a less negative value causes conduction velocity to slow.

Depolarization

Depolarization is the process by which the inside of the cell becomes less negative (Fig. 2-2). This can occur slowly or rapidly, depending on how fast the cell loses its intracellular negativity.

A cell depolarizes according to its type because of one of the following mechanisms:

1. A rapid influx of Na^+ into the cell (atrial and ventricular muscle cells)
2. A slow time-dependent decrease in potassium (K^+) permeability and increase in Na^+ permeability, followed by a rapid influx of Na^+ (cells of the His-Purkinje system)
3. A slow inward calcium (Ca^{++}) and possible Na^+ current (sinus and AV nodal cells)[1-3]

Threshold potential

Threshold potential is a level of membrane potential to which cells must depolarize before they can generate a propagating action potential. For the Purkinje system this is about −70 mV. When this value of negativity is reached, there will be a rapid depolarization until the cell is +30 mV on the inside with respect to the outside. Such a rapid depolarization is then propagated to neighboring cells, causing a current to flow longitudinally through the fiber.

Repolarization

Repolarization is that process by which a cell returns to its resting level of negativity. This is diagrammatically illustrated in Fig. 2-3. Repolarization in cardiac cells is initially rapid and brief, followed by a plateau and again a

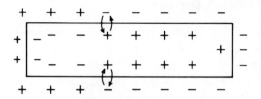

Fig. 2-3. Repolarization.

rapid but longer repolarization to bring the cell to its resting level. This process is explained more fully in the discussion of pacemaker cells.

Sodium-potassium pumps

The resting membrane potential depends on maintenance of a gradient of Na$^+$ to K$^+$ across the cell membrane. A mechanism actively pumps Na$^+$ to the outside of the cell and K$^+$ to the inside. These pumps function in an *electrogenic* fashion; that is, more Na$^+$ is pumped out than K$^+$ is pumped in. The result is a disparity of charge across the membrane.[3]

Pacemaker cells

Fig. 2-4 diagrammatically illustrates the cycle of a pacemaker cell from its resting state, *A*, which is maintained by the ionic pumps, *B*, to the slow diastolic depolarization of the cell, *C*, which culminates in rapid depolarization, *D*, and then repolarizes, *E*, and returns to its resting state, *F*. Following is the explanation of these events:

Pacemaker cells are capable of self-initiated depolarization (automaticity) because of their unstable resting membrane potential. During diastole the pacemaker cell becomes less and less negative (slow diastolic depolarization) until a threshold potential of approximately −60 mV is reached and rapid depolarization ensues. Atrial and ventricular muscle cells do not possess this property of automaticity. They are normally depolarized rapidly because they are driven to threshold by the impulse propagated from the pacemaker cells.

Slow diastolic depolarization is thought to result as the cell becomes less permeable to K$^+$ and more permeable to Na$^+$ (Fig. 2-4, *C*). If K$^+$ cannot leave the cell and more Na$^+$ diffuses in as well, a buildup of positive ions occurs intracellularly, making the cell less negative. When threshold is reached, Na$^+$ rushes into the cell, initiating an action potential (Fig. 2-4, *D*). After this rapid depolarization of the cell, repolarization commences immediately; at first rapidly, then more slowly due to an influx of Ca^{++}, and again rapidly due

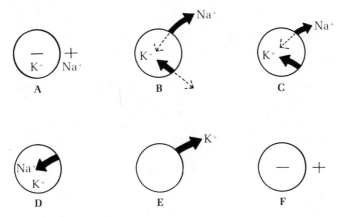

Fig. 2-4. A, Pacemaker cell at rest. **B,** Ionic pumps and membrane conductivity maintain resting membrane potential. **C,** Fall in outward K^+ current causes slow diastolic depolarization. **D,** Depolarization; a threshold is reached and Na^+ rushes in. The sodium pump is inactive. **E,** Potassium rapidly leaves the cell to bring about the completion of repolarization. **F,** Cell returned to its resting state. Black arrows signify active pumps (transport systems). Dotted arrows signify passive currents.

to an exodus of K^+ (Fig. 2-6, E). As the membrane potential returns to its resting state (Fig. 2-6, F), the Na^+-K^+ pump mechanism is reinstated, and the process of self-excitation begins again with a slow buildup of positive ions inside the cell.

The pacemaker cells of the sinus node and nodal-His (NH) region and the nonpacemaker cells of the AV node are thought to depolarize because of a slow inward flux of Ca^{++}. In these cells the resting membrane potential is also lower, and conduction is slow.[1]

Control of the heart rhythm belongs to the pacemaker with the highest level of automaticity. Normally this is the sinus node. However, specialized cardiac cells capable of self-excitation are found throughout the conductive system except for the AV node. The pacemaker cells below the sinus node are called latent pacemakers, since under normal conditions their function is suppressed by the sinus node.

Action potential of ventricular myocardial cells

The action potential consists of depolarization and repolarization. With microelectrodes it is possible to record the action potential, which lasts 100 to 500 msec and is divided into four phases. Fig. 2-5 illustrates the phases of the action potential of a ventricular myocardial cell and the relationship of the action potential to the ECG.

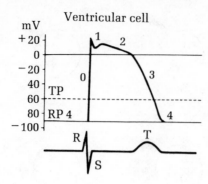

Fig. 2-5. Action potential. *TP*, Threshold potential; *RP*, resting potential.

PHASE 0

The upstroke of the action potential is known as phase 0 (Fig. 2-5) and represents the rapid depolarization of the cell. When a threshold potential is reached due to an applied stimulus or to a stimulus received from a neighboring cell, there is a sudden change in cellular membrane permeability. Na^+ then rushes into the cell, causing a reversal of potential (the cell that was negative on the inside now becoming positive), and produces the upstroke of the action potential.

PHASE 1

Phase 1 is the initial stage of repolarization. This brief, rapid initiation of the repolarization process is believed to be due to an influx of chloride, a negative ion, as well as to an inactivation of the inward Na^+ current.

PHASE 2

During approximately the next 10 msec the repolarization process slows down, causing a plateau (phase 2) in the action potential. This plateau, which does not occur in skeletal muscle, allows the cardiac muscle a more sustained contraction and is thought to be the result of a complex interaction of a slow inward current (predominantly Ca^{++}) with a slow outward K^+ current.

PHASE 3

During phase 3 there is a sudden acceleration in the rate of repolarization as the outward K^+ current increases and the slow Ca^{++} current is inactivated.

PHASE 4

Phase 4 diastolic depolarization distinguishes pacemaker cells from nonpacemaker cells. The *pacemaker cell* has the property of self-excitation. The nonpacemaker cell does not. In Fig. 2-5 note that phase 4 in the pacemaker cell slopes up to a less negative potential until a threshold is reached at approximately −60 mV. The slow diastolic depolarization is caused by a time-

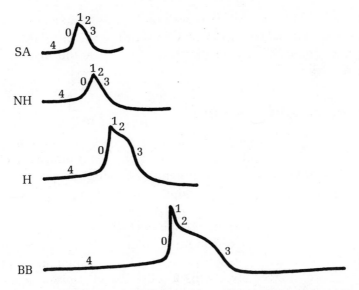

Fig. 2-6. Action potentials of four types of pacemaker cells. *SA,* Sinoatrial, or sinus node; *NH,* nodal His; *H,* bundle of His; *BB,* terminal fascicles of the bundle branches.

dependent fall in outward K^+ current. This, combined with an increase in Na^+ influx, causes a threshold to be reached. Depolarization is thus self-initiated in the pacemaker cells. This process is usually more rapid in the cells of the sinus node, which depolarize first and discharge the lower pacemaker cells before they have a chance to reach threshold on their own. The atrial and ventricular cells reach threshold potential more abruptly, since they are dependent on the pacemaker cells for their depolarization.

Action potential of different types of pacemaker cells

Fig. 2-6 illustrates the action potentials of four types of pacemaker cells. Notice that the cells from the sinus node have the steepest phase 4, causing them to reach threshold potential sooner than do other pacemaker cells. This is why the sinus node dominates the normal cardiac rhythm. Subsidiary pacemakers are capable of reaching threshold on their own but are normally depolarized by an impulse generated in the sinus node.

Note that the action potentials from the SA and NH regions are similar and that they do not have the rapid upstroke of those of the H and BB regions. However, all four share the property of slow diastolic depolarization (self-excitation).

The automatic firing of all pacemaker cells is controlled primarily by the autonomic nervous system and secondarily by changes in cell environment

(K^+, pH, Po_2, and Ca^{++}), as well as by the frequency of stimulation. Suppressed pacemaker cells have a slower diastolic depolarization as the rate of the dominant pacemaker increases. This phenomenon is referred to as *overdrive suppression*.

Membrane responsiveness

The term *membrane responsiveness* refers to the relationship of the resting membrane potential at excitation to the maximum rate of depolarization during phase 0 of the action potential. Conduction velocity and ability of the cardiac muscle fiber to respond to a stimulus are affected if these factors are changed.

The normal resting membrane potential is usually −85 to −90 mV. The higher the level of this membrane potential (the more negativity within the cell), the quicker the rate of depolarization during phase 0 and the higher its amplitude. Conversely, as the level of the membrane potential (voltage) is lowered, so also are the rate of depolarization during phase 0 and its amplitude. Since conduction velocity is directly dependent on these two factors, conduction is also slowed. At about −70 mV conduction disturbance begins to appear. Complete block and lack of response appear at about −55 mV.

Many of the antiarrhythmic agents affect membrane responsiveness by their ability to change either the level of the threshold potential or the duration of the action potential. A change in either of these mechanisms affects the duration of the effective refractory period.

Refractory periods and supernormal period

The *effective refractory period* extends from phase 0 (rapid depolarization) to the point of approximately −50 to −60 mV in the repolarization process. During this time, excitation of the cardiac fiber will not result in propagation of an action potential.

The *relative refractory period* corresponds to the time when the fiber is excitable, but a stronger current is needed to induce a propagated impulse. Also, because of a lower resting membrane potential, conduction velocity from a propagated impulse is markedly slowed. This period extends from the end of the effective refractory period to near the end of repolarization, and corresponds to the second half of the T wave of the ECG.

"*Supernormal*" *period* is the term given to the last part of the repolarization phase before the fiber returns to its resting potential. It is so named because a weaker stimulus delivered to the myocardium at this time can

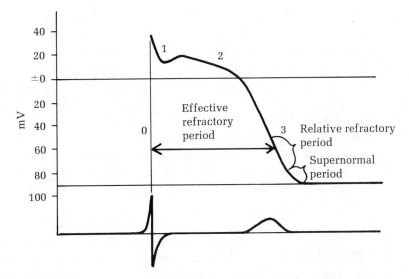

Fig. 2-7. Refractory periods and supernormal period in relation to the ECG.

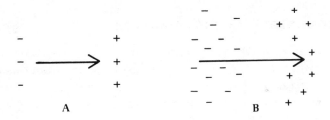

Fig. 2-8. A, Few cells and a small vector. **B,** Many cells and a large vector.

initiate an action potential. The supernormal period corresponds to the latter portion of the T wave.

Vectors

A vector is a physical force (such as current) having both direction and magnitude. A current always flows from negative (depolarized) to positive (polarized) tissue. This current flow is symbolized by an arrow. The length of the arrow indicates the size (amplitude) of the vector force (strength of the current). The point of the arrow indicates the direction of current flow.

In vector *A* of Fig. 2-8 there are only a few negative and a few positive charges. This represents a thin muscle with few cells and therefore a small current. The electrical potential between these two areas is only slight. Therefore the arrow is short.

Vector *B* represents a thicker muscle mass with more cells. The number of negative and positive charges is greater. Therefore the current is greater. A longer arrow is drawn to indicate this greater electrical potential between the two areas. Note that in both examples the current flows from a negative to a positive area.

Briefly, then:

1. The length of each arrow indicates the strength of the current (vector) between the negative and positive areas.
2. This potential in turn depends on the total amount of polarization and depolarization present.
3. The direction of current flow is indicated by an arrow.
4. The point of the arrow represents the positive end of the vector.
5. The length of the arrow represents the strength of the vector.

The atrial vector (current generated during atrial depolarization) is relatively small, since fewer cells are involved. The ventricular vector is much larger, since it is the depolarization of the thick ventricular muscle mass.

Instant-to-instant cardiac vectors

Not all regions of the heart are undergoing depolarization or repolarization at the same instant. Both processes spread from one heart region to another during a single cardiac cycle. The instant-to-instant vectors resulting from the sequential depolarization of the ventricular muscle mass are represented in Fig. 2-9.

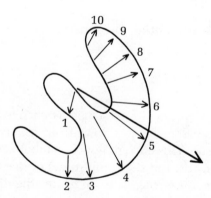

Fig. 2-9. Instant-to-instant vectors resulting from the orderly depolarization of the ventricular muscle mass. The prominent arrow between vectors 5 and 6 represents the mean vector (sum of all the instant-to-instant vectors).

The sum of all the instant-to-instant vectors is referred to as the mean vector (Fig. 2-9). The direction that the mean vector takes is the electrical axis of the heart.

Electrical axis of the heart

In the normal heart, current flows primarily from the base to the apex. It flows from the depolarized (negative) cells to the polarized (positive) cells.

This preponderant direction of current flow in the heart is known as the axis. It is expressed only as a direction, not as a magnitude. The determination of the electrical axis of the heart is covered in Chapter 4.

Summary

Myocardial depolarization is possible because of an ionic imbalance across the cell membranes. The resting membrane potential is dependent on this ionic imbalance and determines the rate of rise and the amplitude of the action potential, which in turn determines conduction velocity. Depolarization and repolarization are two divisions of the action potential; depolarization represents a reversal potential (exchange of ions), and repolarization represents a return to the original potential (another exchange of ions). This is a cyclic process in pacemaker cells because of the fall in outward K^+ current and the increased Na^+ influx that trigger rapid depolarization. The pacemaker cells of the sinus node cycle faster than other pacemaker cells so that the sinus node dominates the heart.

An action potential reached in one cell of the myocardium is propagated to all myocardial cells. This propagation (flow) is a current, or vector, that is cyclic according to heart rate and is usually identical in direction and magnitude each time. The axis of the heart is the main direction that this current takes.

References

1. Cranefield, P. F.: The conduction of the cardiac impulse: the slow response and cardiac arrhythmias, New York, 1975, Futura Publishing Co.
2. Cranefield, P. F.: Action potentials, afterpotentials, and arrhythmias, Circ. Res. **41**:415, 1977.
3. Rosen, M. R., and Danilo, P.: The electrophysiological basis for cardiac arrhythmias. In Narula, O. S., editor: Electrophysiology, diagnosis and management, Baltimore, 1979, The Williams & Wilkins Co.

CHAPTER 3

Arrhythmogenesis

Normally the heart is paced by the spontaneous activity of the sinus node at a regular rate consistent with the physiological demands of the body. The automatic impulse generated in the sinus node normally dominates all the fibers of the heart. When this rhythm is disturbed or usurped or its conduction interfered with, the term *arrhythmia* or *dysrhythmia* is used.

Since 1954 it has been known that there are two main electrophysiological arrhythmogenic mechanisms in myocardial infarction.[1] Later evidence proved these two mechanisms to be reentry and enhanced automaticity. It was shown that reentry is responsible for the arrhythmias in the first few hours after coronary occlusion[2-5] and that enhanced automaticity causes the arrhythmias occurring 4 to 24 hours after occlusion.[6,7] Recently another arrhythmogenic mechanism has been described: afterdepolarization as a cause of *triggered activity*.[8-11]

In this chapter these mechanisms and the resultant arrhythmias will be discussed. On the surface ECG it is often impossible to distinguish one mechanism from another. It is especially difficult to distinguish between the paroxysmal ventricular tachycardia and coupled beats that result from reentry and those that result from afterdepolarization. However, future research may help in this regard, and specific therapy may depend on a precise understanding of electrophysiological arrhythmogenic mechanisms.

Circus reentry

Circus reentry refers to that condition in which a cardiac impulse is delayed long enough within a pathway of slow conduction that it is still active when the surrounding myocardium repolarizes. The impulse can then *reenter* the surrounding tissue and produce another propagated impulse.

Slow conduction may result whenever depolarization occurs at a decreased membrane potential. Among the causes of a decreased resting membrane potential are ischemia and hyperkalemia. Also, a stimulus occurring during phase 3 of the action potential finds cells with a lower membrane potential and hence slow conduction. Thus a beat occurring during the T wave of the ECG has a slow impulse propagation and may support a reentry tachycardia or precipitate fibrillation.

Conditions necessary for a reentry circuit to be established follow[12-14]:

1. An initiating impulse, either normal sinus or ectopic
2. An area of slow conduction that is sufficiently long and/or slow for the impulse passing through it to still be active when the rest of the myocardium has become nonrefractory
3. One-way block, without which the impulse would cancel itself out within the area of slow conduction

Any part of the myocardium or conductive network may support reentry as long as the above conditions are met. In the discussion to follow, reentry through the following structures will be considered: isolated Purkinje fibers and His-Purkinje system (intraventricular), AV node, sinus node, and intra-atrial via the internodal or interatrial tracts. Reentry through anomalous pathways (preexcitation syndrome) will be discussed in Chapter 11.

INTRAVENTRICULAR REENTRY

Reentry through a microcircuit in the Purkinje system has been thought to be the mechanism responsible for the life-threatening ventricular arrhythmias in the first few hours after coronary occlusion.[2-5,15,16] This type of reentry is thought to produce coupled ventricular extrasystoles,[8] that is, extrasystoles that are always exactly linked to the preceding normal complex. Such a reentry circuit may also support a paroxysm of ventricular tachycardia.

In 1974 Akhtar et al. described a macrocircuit involving the bundle of His, right and left bundle branches, and ventricular myocardium.[17]

Microreentry. Fig. 3-1, B, illustrates a microreentry circuit within the Purkinje system. Note the area of depressed conduction and one-way block (shaded area). A normal ventricular excitation wave (producing a normal complex) may be conducted slowly through such an area in one direction only and recapture the rest of the myocardium after it has repolarized. If the conduction time through the shaded area remains the same for each beat, the abnormal complex always follows the normal one at exactly the same time interval, resulting in what is called *fixed coupling* and a bigeminal rhythm.

Macroreentry. Fig. 3-1, C, illustrates a postulated macroreentry circuit[17] involving both bundle branches, the bundle of His, and the ventricular myocardium. Such a circuit was found to produce a single reentrant beat and was initiated by a ventricular ectopic beat, which itself was closely coupled to the preceding beat. Note in Fig. 3-1, C, the area of depressed conduction (shaded area) and the retrograde block in one of the bundle branches. If the impulse is in transit long enough through the depressed bundle branch, it could then arrive at the bundle of His when the other bundle branch (previously blocked) is nonrefractory and be conducted antegradely with bundle branch block, since the depressed bundle branch that initially conducted

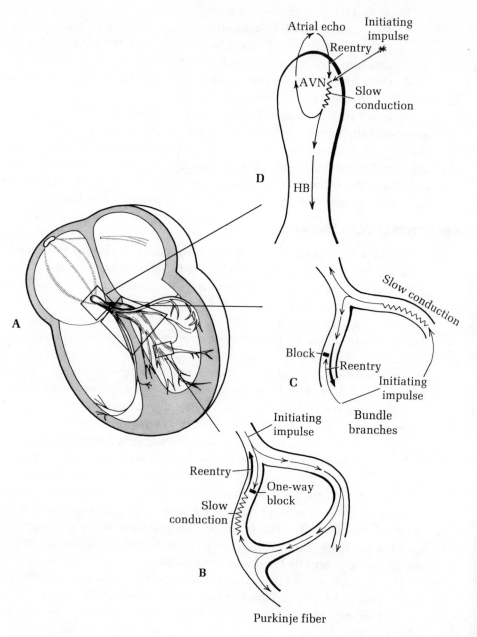

Fig. 3-1. A, Reentry circuit involving the following structures: isolated Purkinje fibers and His-Purkinje system, (intraventricular), AV node (internodal), sinus node, and internodal or inter-arterial tracts. **B,** Microreentry. **C,** Macroreentry. **D,** AV nodal reentry. *AVN,* AV node; *HB,* His bundle.

would now be refractory. Such a circuit was not found to support more than one or two extra beats.

AV NODAL REENTRY

Reentry through the AV node has gained wide acceptance as the cause of many paroxysmal supraventricular tachycardias, excluding Wolff-Parkinson-White syndrome.[18-25]

Such a reentry circuit presupposes two pathways within the AV node, one conducting slowly and the other more rapidly. A critically timed atrial stimulus passes antegradely down the slow pathway and retrogradely up the more rapid pathway. This return current to the atria produces what is called an atrial echo beat. If the circuit is sustained, antegrade conduction to the ventricles (again, through the slow path) produces what is called a reciprocal beat, and so on, with alternating atrial echo and ventricular reciprocal beats. Hence the resulting tachycardia is sometimes termed a *reciprocating tachycardia*. Fig. 3-1, *D*, illustrates an AV nodal reentry circuit. AV nodal reciprocating tachycardia is further illustrated and discussed on pp. 86 to 87.

AV nodal reentry may also be initiated by a premature junctional beat or a ventricular ectopic beat with retrograde conduction to the atria.

SINUS NODE REENTRY

Reentry through the sinus node has been reported to be another cause of paroxysmal supraventricular tachycardia.[26-30] In such a case a critically timed atrial premature beat would be conducted slowly and in only one direction through the sinus node and perinodal tissue, arriving in atrial tissue after it has repolarized, thus producing an atrial echo beat. Such an atrial excitation has a P wave that is identical in morphology to the normal sinus P wave and thus may mimic a paroxysmal sinus tachycardia.

INTRA-ATRIAL REENTRY

In the atria a circus reentry pathway could be provided by the anatomical distribution of the specialized internodal and interatrial tracts. There is some evidence to support intra-atrial reentry as a mechanism of paroxysmal supraventricular tachycardia.[30,31] Intra-atrial reentry is also a possible mechanism for atrial flutter, although the basic mechanism of this arrhythmia remains unknown.

Focal reentry

When neighboring fibers are activated simultaneously or almost simultaneously and yet repolarize at different rates, a second beat may be initiated. This phenomenon is called focal reentry and occurs when the already repolarized fibers are reexcited by fibers that are still repolarizing. The extra beat generated is closely coupled to the preceding complex. In dog ventricles it has been shown that this disparity in refractory periods is increased by ischemia, sympathetic stimulation, hypokalemia, toxic doses of ouabain, premature beats, chloroform, quinidine, and hypothermia. Reentry and ventricular fibrillation may be produced by any one of these factors.

Altered automaticity
NORMAL AUTOMATICITY REVIEWED

As explained in Chapter 2, pacemaker cells possess the property of self-excitation. The working (contracting) cells in the atria or ventricles do not. The electrophysiological difference between the two types of cells lies in the fact that pacemaker cells have an unstable membrane potential during phase 4. The transmembrane potential decreases to a less negative value until a threshold is reached and rapid depolarization ensues (phase 0). Nonpacemaker cells maintain a stable resting potential (phase 4) until the next propagated impulse arrives and causes rapid depolarization. Nonpacemaker cells are therefore dependent on pacemaker cells for their excitation.

Cells demonstrating the property of slow diastolic depolarization are said to be automatic. Control of the heart rhythm belongs to the sinus node because it possesses the highest level of automaticity; that is, the cells in the sinus node reach a threshold potential sooner than is normally possible in the lower pacemaker cells, although the latter would manifest this property if the sinus node failed to dominate.

The sinus node pacemaker, by dominating all subsidiary pacemakers, depresses their automaticity so that there is less likelihood that a lower pacemaker will interfere with the regular normal function of the sinus node. This phenomenon is called overdrive suppression and was discussed in Chapter 2. Disease and the action of some drugs can negate and even reverse overdrive suppression. For example, catecholamines and digitalis in toxic doses enhance automaticity and increase the likelihood of ectopic rhythms.

The rate of automaticity is controlled primarily by the autonomic nervous system and secondarily by cell environment (p. 220).

ENHANCED AUTOMATICITY

If there is an acceleration of phase 4 (Fig. 3-2) in the latent pacemaker cells (those below the sinus node), automaticity is enhanced and premature ectopic beats may occur. These may be single ectopic beats (atrial, junctional, or ventricular premature beats), or a sustained ectopic rhythm (atrial,[33] ventricular,[6,7] or junctional tachycardia[32]).

Some of the causes of acceleration of slow diastolic depolarization (phase 4) follow: hypoxia, stretch of the conductive fibers, hypokalemia, hypocal-

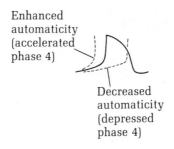

Enhanced
automaticity
(accelerated
phase 4)

Decreased
automaticity
(depressed
phase 4)

Fig. 3-2. Action potential of a pacemaker cell. The dark line represents a normal phase 4. The broken lines represent an *accelerated* and a *depressed phase 4*, respectively.

cemia, heat, trauma, hypercapnia, catecholamines, digitalis toxicity, and atropine.

DECREASED AUTOMATICITY

Retardation of phase 4 (Fig. 3-2) causes depressed automaticity and results in bradycardia and escape rhythms.

Some of the causes of deceleration of the process of slow diastolic depolarization follow: vagal stimulation, ischemia, a sudden increase in local extracellular K^+, decreased catecholamines, quinidine, procainamide (Pronestyl), propranolol (Inderal), edrophonium chloride (Tensilon), acetylcholine, and hypothermia.

Afterdepolarization and triggered activity [8,9,11,12]

The term *triggered activity* has been coined by Cranefield to refer to repetitive ectopic firing that is not the result of enhanced automaticity and is not sustained by circus movement reentry. It is rather the result of a previous impulse.

Triggered activity has recently been described as originating from non-pacemaker cells as well as from pacemaker cells and is the result of a slower type of depolarization (inward positive current) occurring after the well-known rapid Na^+ influx depolarization (p. 15). This slow inward current is thought to be mainly Ca^{++}. The depolarization it causes has been called *afterdepolarization*, since it occurs only after either a driven or an automatic action potential.

Some causes of such a slow depolarizing current include catecholamines, digitalis, hypoxia, injury, stretch, cooling, barium (Ba^{++}), and veratrine.

Afterdepolarizations can occur rhythmically without producing extrasystoles or ectopic tachycardias if threshold potential is not reached and thus may not be manifest on the ECG as ectopic beats or rhythms. Some reasons

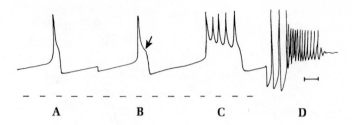

Fig. 3-3. A, Normal action potential. **B,** Early afterdepolarization (arrow). **C,** Four nondriven action potentials occur at a membrane potential corresponding to that of the early afterdepolarization. **D,** Three normal action potentials, followed by a train of activity at a low membrane potential, followed by quiescence. (From Cranefield, P. F.: Action potentials, afterpotentials, and arrhythmias, Circ. Res. **41:**415, 1977. By permission of the American Heart Association, Inc.)

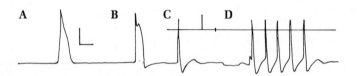

Fig. 3-4. A, Normal action potential. **B,** Early afterhyperpolarization. **C,** Early afterhyperpolarization, followed by a delayed afterdepolarization. **D,** A driven action potential, followed by four nondriven action potentials that arise from delayed afterdepolarization. (From Cranefield, P. F.: Action potentials, afterpotentials, and arrhythmias, Circ. Res. **41:**415, 1977. By permission of the American Heart Association, Inc.)

why the afterdepolarization reaches threshold are an increase in heart rate, catecholamines, or a premature ectopic beat. Agents that reduce the amplitude of the afterdepolarization are manganese (Mn^+), verapamil, and D-600, which is like verapamil in action.

Clinically, the afterdepolarization that reaches threshold potential produces a paroxysm of atrial or ventricular ectopic tachycardia or coupled ectopic beats, which cannot be differentiated (1) from the paroxysm of tachycardia that is initiated by enhanced automaticity and sustained by a reentry circuit or (2) from the coupled extrasystole that may result from reentry.

The mechanism sustaining the burst of tachycardia that results from triggered activity follows: when at least one action potential, driven or automatic, is followed by an afterdepolarization of sufficient amplitude to reach threshold, the resulting action potential may then itself be followed by another afterdepolarization, producing another nondriven action potential, and so on.

Afterdepolarizations are illustrated in Figs. 3-3 and 3-4. They may be either early or delayed. The early afterdepolarization interrupts repolarization (Fig. 3-3). The delayed afterdepolarization (Fig. 3-4) occurs after repolarization is completed.

Summary

Myocardial ischemia, various drugs, and other factors may upset the electrophysiological and ionic balance of the myocardium so that (1) automaticity is altered, (2) conduction velocity is decreased, (3) refractory periods in different parts of the heart are not the same, and/or (4) afterdepolarizations exist that may cause triggered activity.

Enhanced automaticity causes premature ectopic beats and rhythms. Reentry may result from decreased conduction velocity (circus reentry) or dispersion of refractory periods (focal reentry), producing premature ectopic beats and rhythms. Afterdepolarization may be the result of digitalis excess, ischemia, catecholamines, or an abrupt change in cycle length. Such an afterpotential may produce a burst of tachycardia (atrial or ventricular).

Reentry may occur through the Purkinje network, His-Purkinje system, AV node, sinus node, or intra-atrial conductive system.

References

GENERAL

1. Harris, A. S., Bisteni, A., Russel, R. A., Brigham, J. C., and Firestone, J. E.: Excitatory factors in ventricular tachycardia resulting from myocardial ischemia. Potassium a major excitant, Science **119**:200, 1954.
2. Scherlag, B. J., Helfant, R. H., Haft, J. I., and Damato, A. N.: Electrophysiology underlying ventricular arrhythmias due to coronary ligation, Am. J. Physiol. **219**:1665, 1969.
3. Cox, J. L., Danile, T. M., Sabiston, D. C. and Boineau, J. P.: Desynchronized activation in myocardial infarction: a reentry basis for ventricular arrhythmias (abstr.), Circulation **39**(supp. 3):63, 1969.
4. Gambetta, M., and Childers, R. W.: Initial electrophysiologic disturbance in experimental myocardial infarction (abstr.), Ann. Intern. Med. **70**:1076, 1969.
5. Han, J.: Mechanisms of ventricular arrhythmias associated with myocardial infarction, Am. J. Cardiol. **24**:800, 1969.
6. Scherlag, B. J., Lazzara, R., Abelleira, J. L., and Samet, P.: Mechanisms of early and late arrhythmias due to myocardial ischemia and infarction (abstr.), Circulation **46**(supp. 2):59, 1972.
7. Lazzara, R., El-Sherif, N., and Scherlag, B. J.: Electrophysiological properties of canine Purkinje cells in one-day-old myocardial infarction, Circ. Res. **33**:722, 1973.

MICROREENTRY AND TRIGGERED ACTIVITY

8. Cranefield, P. F.: The conduction of the cardiac impulse; the slow response and cardiac

arrhythmias, New York, 1975, Futura Publishing Co.
9. Cranefield, P. F.: Action potentials, afterpotentials, and arrhythmias, Circ. Res. **41**:415, 1977.
10. Wit, A. L., Bigger, J. T.: Possible electrophysiological mechanisms for lethal arrhythmias accompanying myocardial ischemia and infarction, Circulation **51**(supp. 3):96, 1975.
11. Rosen, M. R., and Danilo, P.: The electrophysiological basis for cardiac arrhythmias. In Narula, O. S., editor: Cardiac arrhythmias: electrophysiology, diagnosis and management, Baltimore, 1979, The Williams & Wilkins Co.
12. Wit, A. L., Boyden, G. A., Gadsby, D. C., and Cranefield, P. F.: Triggered activity as a cause of atrial arrhythmias. In Narula, O. S., editor: Cardiac arrhythmias: electrophysiology, diagnosis and management, Baltimore, 1979, The Williams & Wilkins Co.
13. Cranefield, P. F., Klein, H. O., and Hoffman, B. R.: Conduction of the cardiac impulse. Delay, block and one-way block in depressed Purkinje fibers, Circ. Res. **28**:199, 1971.
14. Wit, A. L., Hoffman, B. F., and Cranefield, P. F.: Slow conduction and reentry in the ventricular conducting system, Circ. Res. **30**:1, 1972.

MACROREENTRY

15. Singer, D. H., Lazzara, R., and Hoffman, B. R.: Interrelationship between automatic-

ity and conduction in Purkinje fibers, Circ. Res. **21**:537, 1967.

16. Watanabe, Y., and Dreifus, L. S.: Newer concepts in the genesis of cardiac arrhythmias, Am. Heart J. **76**:114, 1968.

17. Akhtar, M., Damato, A. N., Batsford, W. P., Ruskin, J. N., Ogunkelu, J. B., and Vargas, G.: Demonstration of re-entry within the His-Purkinje system in man, Circulation **50**:1150, 1974.

AV NODAL REENTRY

18. Janse, M. J., Van Capelle, F. J. L., Freud, G. E., and Durrer, D.: Circus movement within the A-V node as a basis for supraventricular tachycardia as shown by multiple microelectrode recording in the isolated rabbit heart, Circ. Res. **28**:403, 1971.

19. Bigger, J. T. Jr., and Goldreyer, B. N.: The mechanism of paroxysmal supraventricular tachycardia, Circulation **42**:673, 1970.

20. Goldreyer, B. N., and Bigger, J. T., Jr.: The site of reentry in paroxysmal supraventricular tachycardia, Circulation **43**:15, 1971.

21. Goldreyer, B. N., and Damato, A. N.: The essential role of A-V conduction delay in the initiation of paroxysmal supraventricular tachycardia, Circulation **43**:679, 1971.

22. Wit, A. L., Goldreyer, B. N., and Damato, A. N.: In vitro model of paroxysmal supraventricular tachycardia, Circulation **43**:862, 1971.

23. Moe, G. K., Preston, G. B., and Burlington, H.: Physiologic evidence for a dual AV transmission system, Circ. Res. **4**:357, 1956.

24. Wellens, H. J. J.: Electrical stimulation of the heart in the study and treatment of tachycardias, Baltimore, 1971, University Park Press.

25. Barold, S. S., and Coumel, P.: Mechanisms of atrioventricular junctional tachycardia. Role of reentry and concealed accessory bypass tracts, Am. J. Cardiol. **39**:97, 1977.

SINUS NODE REENTRY

26. Han, J., Malazzi, A. M., and Moe, G. K.: Sinoatrial reciprocation in the isolated rabbit heart, Circ. Res. **22**:355, 1968.

27. Narula, O. S.: Sinus node re-entry, Circulation **50**:1114, 1974.

28. Narula, O. S.: Sinus node re-entry. Mechanism of supraventricular tachycardia (SVT) in man, Circulation **46**(supp. 2):27, 1972.

29. Pauley, L. L., Varghese, P. J., and Damato, A. N.: Sinus node re-entry: an in vivo demonstration in the dog, Circ. Res. **32**:455, 1973.

INTRA-ATRIAL REENTRY

30. Wu, D., Amat-y-Leon, F., Denes, P., et al.: Demonstration of sustained sinus and atrial reentry as a mechanism of paroxysmal supraventricular tachycardia, Circulation **51**:234, 1975.

31. Ogawa, S., Dreifus, L. S., and Osmick, M. J.: Longitudinal dissociation of Bachmann's bundle as a mechanism of paroxysmal supraventricular tachycardia, Am. J. Cardiol. **40**:915, 1977.

ENHANCED AUTOMATICITY

32. Rosen, K. M.: Junctional tachycardia: mechanisms, diagnosis, differential diagnosis, and management, Circulation **47**:654, 1973.

33. Goldreyer, B. N., Gallagher, J. J., and Damato, A. N.: The electrophysiologic demonstration of atrial ectopic tachycardia in man, Am. Heart J. **85**:205, 1973.

CHAPTER 4

Determination of electrical axis

A lead and its axis defined

A bipolar lead is composed of two electrodes, one positive and one negative, or one electrode and a reference point. An imaginary line drawn between these two electrodes, or between an electrode and the reference point, is known as the axis of the lead.

Electrocardiography and its functions

The heart is an electrical field in which currents flow in repetitive patterns according to the heart rate. These currents can be detected at the level of the skin with two electrodes of opposite polarity that are placed at opposite poles of the electrical field. The electrodes are attached to an amplifier within an oscilloscope or strip recorder. These instruments then accurately record the electrical events of the heart: direction of current flow and magnitude of the current. The interpretation of these events is the basis for the electrocardiographic diagnosis of arrhythmias and cardiac disease.

DIRECTION OF CURRENT FLOW

Direction of current flow is indicated in the following manner: a current flowing toward the positive terminal of the lead axis is recorded as a positive (upright) deflection. A current directed toward the negative terminal of the lead axis is recorded as a negative (downward) deflection. A current directed exactly perpendicular to the lead axis records a net zero potential because both electrodes sense exactly the same force. This is indicated by a deflection that is equal in both directions.

MAGNITUDE OF CURRENT

The strength of the vector is indicated by the recording of a small deflection for a weak vector and a large deflection for a strong vector.

Bipolar leads

The bipolar leads compare the electrical potentials between two electrode (− and +) terminals. The axis of the lead is determined by the two electrodes.

The ECG from a bipolar lead is a reflection of the orientation of the cardia vectors to this axis. In the twelve-lead ECG only three of the leads are bipo lar: I,.II, and III.

The arms and legs are linear extensions of the electrical field surroundin the heart. Therefore an electrode placed on the right arm senses the sam electrical potentials that would be sensed at the right shoulder. The sam relationship applies for electrodes on the other extremities.

The axis of lead I extends from shoulder to shoulder. The negative elec trode is on the right arm, and the positive electrode is on the left arm.

The axis of lead II extends from the right shoulder to the left leg or to point just below the left rib cage. The negative electrode is on the right arm and the positive electrode is on the left leg.

The axis of lead III extends from the left shoulder to the left leg or to point just below the left rib cage. The negative electrode is on the left arm and the positive electrode is on the left leg.

EINTHOVEN TRIANGLE

Willem Einthoven, the father of electrocardiography, first introduced the three bipolar limb leads, and thus the triangle they form bears his name The Einthoven triangle is illustrated in Fig. 4-1. Einthoven also arrived at the following equation, known as Einthoven's law:

$$\text{Lead I} + \text{Lead III} + (-\text{lead II}) = 0$$

Or

$$\text{Lead I} + \text{Lead III} = \text{Lead II}$$

Cardiac vectors related to the lead axis

The vector in Fig. 4-2, *A*, would cause a positive deflection to be written for lead I because the flow is toward the positive terminal of the lead axis

The polarity of the deflection in Fig. 4-2, *B*, would be negative, since the current is directed toward the negative terminal of the lead axis.

Figs. 4-3 (lead II) and 4-4 (lead III) illustrate the same principle: when a current flows toward a positive electrode, a positive deflection is inscribed; when a current is oriented toward a negative electrode, a negative deflection is inscribed.

Fig. 4-5 combines a number of mean vectors into one illustration so that the different complexes produced can be compared. When the mean vector is perpendicular to the lead axis, an equiphasic deflection results. An equi- phasic deflection is one that equals zero when the value of the positive and negative components are added. A mean vector that is neither perpendicular nor parallel to the lead axis produces a complex that is somewhere in be-

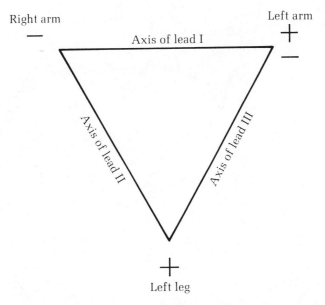

Fig. 4-1. Axes of the 3 standard limb leads form the Einthoven triangle.

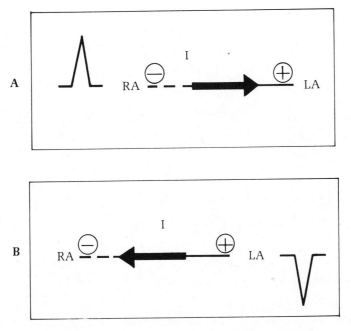

Fig. 4-2. Vectors that are parallel to the axis of lead *I*.

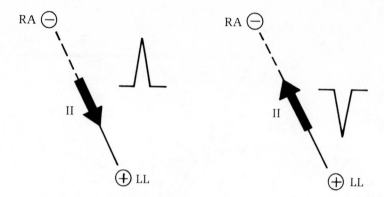

Fig. 4-3. Vectors that are parallel to the axis of lead *II*.

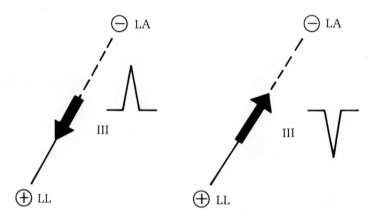

Fig. 4-4. Vectors that are parallel to the axis of lead *III*.

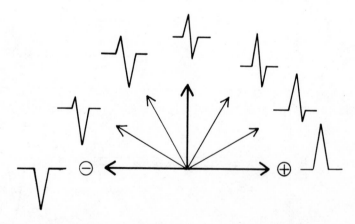

Fig. 4-5. A number of mean vectors are combined here to illustrate the different complexes possible. A mean vector that is perpendicular to the lead axis produces an equiphasic deflection. A mean vector on the positive side of the perpendicular and yet not parallel with the lead axis produces a complex that is mostly positive. However, if the mean vector is on the negative side of the perpendicular and yet not parallel with the lead axis, the complex is mostly negative.

tween equiphasic and fully negative or fully positive, depending on its orientation to the positive electrode.

Note that the tallest positive or deepest negative deflection is inscribed when the mean vector is parallel to the axis of the lead.

nipolar limb leads

There are three unipolar limbs leads: aV_R, aV_L, and aV_F (Fig. 4-6). The letter "a" stands for *augmented*, a term added when it was discovered that by eliminating a negative electrode, the amplitude of the recording is augmented by 50%. "V" indicates a unipolar lead. The inferior capital letters "R," "L," and "F" indicate where the positive electrode is placed—the *r*ight arm, *l*eft arm, and the left leg (*f*oot).

The unipolar lead compares the electrical potentials of the heart with zero. This zero potential is achieved by adding up the electrical potentials from the three bipolar limb leads, which is a point in the center of the electrical field. (See Einthoven's law, p. 34.) Thus the axis of the unipolar lead is an imaginary line drawn from the positive lead site to the center of the heart, as shown in Fig. 4-6.

Note in Fig. 4-7 that the axis of each unipolar limb lead is perpendicular to the axis of a bipolar limb lead. For example, the axis of aV_F is perpendicular to the axis of lead I; likewise aV_R is perpendicular to III and aV_L to II. As will be seen, this gives an excellent reference frame in which to determine the electrical axis of the heart.

An easy two-step method to axis determination
NORMAL AXIS OF THE HEART

The normal axis of the heart is described differently by different authorities, some placing it in the narrow bounds between +30 and +60 degrees (Sodi-Pallares) and others in the quadrant between 0 and +90 degrees (Marriott).

The coronary care nurse is required to determine the electrical axis of the heart because this, plus QRS morphology, is the method of determining hemiblock. Therefore, in this book I have chosen to describe left axis deviation (LAD) as being beyond −30 degrees, right axis deviation (RAD) as being beyond +110 degrees, and a normal axis as being between these (Fig. 4-8).

Note that axis determination is made only from the limb leads. Fig. 4-9 illustrates one possible normal axis (+90 degrees). This can easily be deduced from the fact that there is an equiphasic deflection in lead I, indicating a mean current perpendicular to the axis of that lead. However, this information alone does not indicate whether the current is traveling downward to-

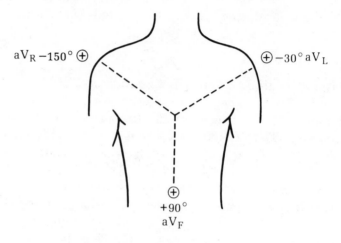

Fig. 4-6. Unipolar limb lead axes.

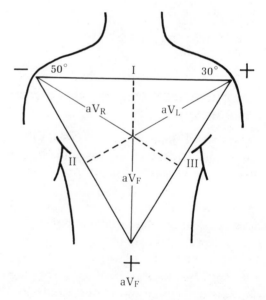

Fig. 4-7. Axes of the 6 limb leads.

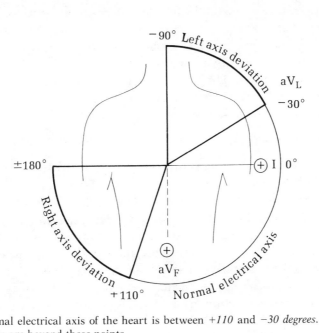

Fig. 4-8. Normal electrical axis of the heart is between *+110* and *−30 degrees*. Right and left axis deviations are beyond these points.

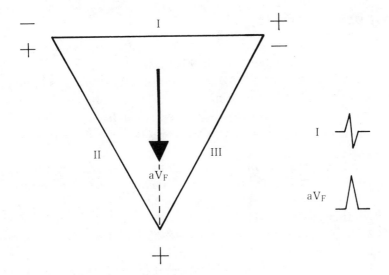

Fig. 4-9. Deflections in I and aV_F when the axis is +90 degrees (normal).

ward +90 or upward toward −90 degrees. Such a determination is easily made by noting that aV_F, the lead axis perpendicular to lead I, is positive, indicating that the mean current is flowing toward the positive electrode of that lead. The current is also flowing toward the positive electrode of leads II and III, which are also upright.

For ease in recognizing a normal axis, it can be stated that leads I and II should normally be upright to equiphasic and never negative. Lead III can normally be any configuration.

LEFT AXIS DEVIATION (LAD)

A deviation of the mean QRS vector beyond −30 degrees to the left is considered abnormal (Fig. 4-8).

Fig. 4-10 illustrates an LAD of −60 degrees. Note that this is easily recognized because there is an equiphasic deflection in lead aV_R, indicating a mean current perpendicular to the axis of that lead. A glance at lead III, the lead axis parallel to the current flow, indicates that the mean current is traveling toward the negative electrode of that lead (−60 degrees).

Generally speaking, for instant recognition LAD always presents with a mainly positive deflection in lead I and a mainly negative deflection in the inferior leads (II, III, and aV_F).

LAD may be a normal variation, or it may be the result left anterior hemiblock, inferior wall myocardial infarction, ventricular tachycardia, or Wolff-Parkinson-White (WPW) syndrome.

RIGHT AXIS DEVIATION (RAD)

When the mean QRS vector is deviated to the right beyond +110 degrees, it is considered abnormal (Fig. 4-8).

Fig. 4-11 illustrates a RAD of +120 degrees. This is easily determined because of the equiphasic deflection in aV_R, indicating a mean current perpendicular to the axis of this lead. Because the deflection in lead III is positive, the mean current is flowing toward the positive electrode of that lead (+120 degrees).

To review: The equiphasic deflection in aV_R indicates only that the mean current is perpendicular to that lead axis. In order to determine if the current is to the right or the left, look at the lead axis that is parallel to the current, in this case lead III. This lead is either strongly positive or strongly negative. In the case illustrated the deflection in lead III is strongly positive, placing the axis at +120 degrees.

Generally speaking, for easy recognition RAD is always mainly negative in lead I and positive in the inferior leads (II, III, and aV_F).

RAD is seen as a normal variation and also in right ventricular hypertrophy, left posterior hemiblock, and Wolff-Parkinson-White syndrome.

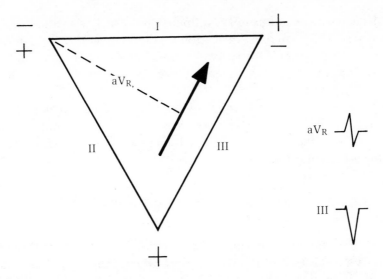

Fig. 4-10. Deflections in aV_R and III when the axis is -60 degrees (LAD).

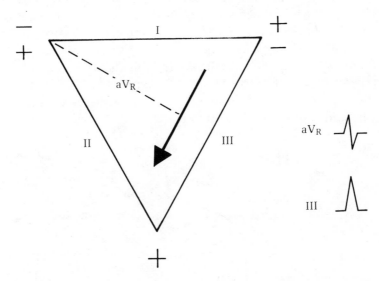

Fig. 4-11. Deflections in aV_R and III when the axis is $+120$ degrees (RAD).

HOW TO PROCEED WITHOUT AN EQUIPHASIC DEFLECTION

In the event that there is not an equiphasic deflection in the six limb leads, a third step is required. Find the smallest deflection and proceed as if it were actually equiphasic; that is, (1) place the axis of the heart as if it were perpendicular to this lead axis and (2) determine which way the current is flowing by looking at the lead axis parallel to the current. Now, (3) since the deflection was not exactly equiphasic in step 1, you must make a small correction. If the smallest deflection was more negative than positive, move the axis of the heart slightly away from the positive electrode. If the deflection was more positive than negative, then move the axis a little toward the positive electrode of that lead.

Once you have become comfortable and adept at determining electrical axis by the above method, you may wish to refine your skill by learning to work with the hexaxial figure, which provides an excellent reference system for estimating the axis in degrees.

The hexaxial figure: a more precise method for axis determination

The triaxial figure (Fig. 4-12) is drawn by shifting the three standard limb lead axes (I, II, and III) so that they all pass through what is considered the zero potential of the heart's electrical field.

When the axes of the three unipolar limb leads are added to this figure, it is called the hexaxial figure (Fig. 4-13). Such a reference figure is particularly useful when one does not find an equiphasic deflection in the limb leads or when the axis happens to be between −90 and 180 degrees. Note that leads I and aV$_F$ divide the electrical field of the heart into quadrants, 0 to 180 degrees horizontally and +90 to −90 degrees vertically. Within each quadrant there are two other lead axes, each having increments of 30 degrees. Thus, when an equiphasic deflection is not present, just look at I and aV$_F$ to place

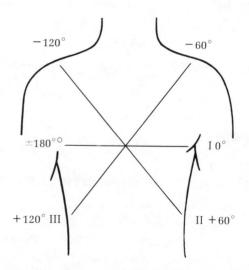

Fig. 4-12. Triaxial figure.

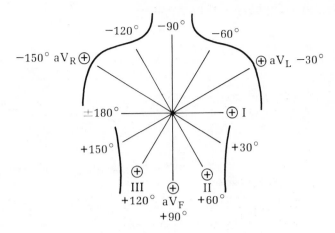

Fig. 4-13. Hexaxial figure illustrating the direction of each limb lead and the location of the positive electrodes.

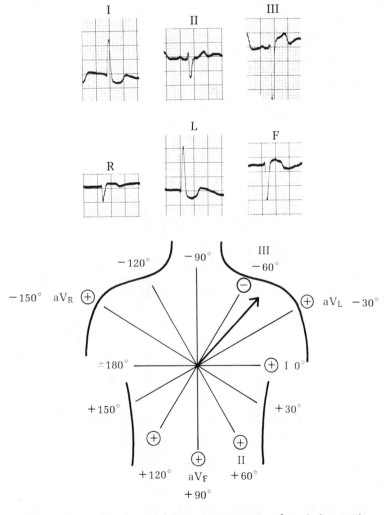

Fig. 4-14. Use of the hexaxial figure in pinpointing the axis (see text).

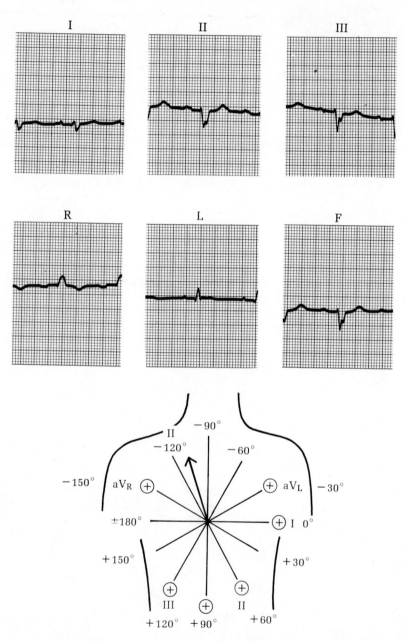

Fig. 4-15. Use of the hexaxial figure in pinpointing the axis (see text).

the axis of the heart in one of the quadrants. Then determine which of the two other leads within that quadrant has the largest complex. For example, in Fig. 4-14, A, no equiphasic deflection is seen in any of the limb leads. However, the axis is easily placed in the upper left quadrant because lead I is positive and aV_F is negative. Now look at III and aV_L, the other two leads within this quadrant. Lead III is more negative than aV_L is positive, placing the main current flow closer to the axis of III than to that of aV_L, or at about -50 degrees (Fig. 4-14, B), an LAD.

Extreme axis deviation

The upper right-hand quadrant is sometimes referred to as *no-man's-land* (between -90 and ±180 degrees). When the axis falls within this quadrant, it may be either extreme right (±180 to -150 degrees) or extreme left axis deviation (-90 to -120 degrees). In Fig. 4-15, A, both I and aV_F are negative, placing the main current flow within the upper right-hand quadrant. Now look at the other two leads within this quadrant (II and aV_R). Lead II is clearly more negative than aV_R is positive, placing the axis closer to II. However, if the axis were parallel with the axis of II, aV_L would be equiphasic. Since this is not the case, aV_L being positive, the axis is approximately midway between -90 and -120 degrees, or -115 degrees (Fig. 4-15, B).

Ventricular tachycardia commonly has an axis in no-man's-land, giving a helpful morphological clue when there is a differential diagnosis between ventricular ectopy and aberration (pp. 143 to 153).

Precordial leads

The chest (precordial) leads are unipolar, that is, each lead consists of one positive electrode and a zero potential reference point, achieved as with

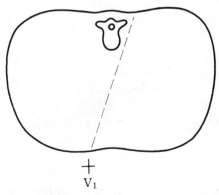

Fig. 4-16. Axes of the precordial leads (horizontal plane).

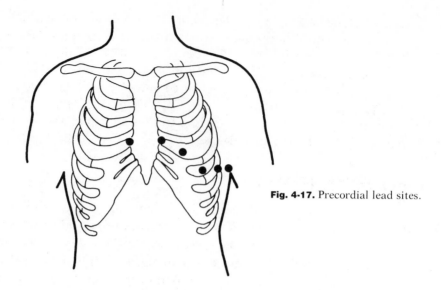

Fig. 4-17. Precordial lead sites.

the unipolar limb leads: $I + III + (-II) = 0$. This zero potential is the center of the heart. The axis of these leads is an imaginary line drawn from the positive electrode to the heart center. The precordial leads are therefore on a horizontal plane and thus give information about anterior and posterior forces, as well as right and left forces.

The normal precordial complexes are illustrated in Chapter 5.

AXIS OF V_1

The positive electrode of V_1 is placed at the fourth intercostal space of the right sternal border. The axis extends from this site to the heart center, as seen in Fig. 4-16.

PRECORDIAL LEAD SITES

The six precordial lead sites (Fig. 4-17) follow:

V_1 Fourth intercostal space, right sternal border
V_2 Fourth intercostal space, left sternal border
V_3 Equidistant between V_2 and V_4
V_4 Fifth intercostal space, left midclavicular line
V_5 Lateral to V_4 at the anterior axillary line
V_6 Lateral to V_5 at the midaxillary line

MCL$_1$

MCL$_1$ is a bipolar lead that stimulates the unipolar precordial lead V_1. (M = modified; C = chest position for positive electrode; L = left arm for

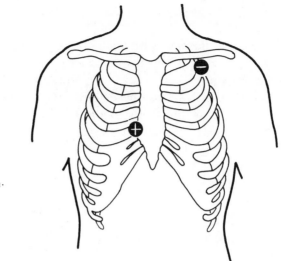

Fig. 4-18. MCL$_1$.

negative electrode.) The positive electrode is placed, as is the electrode for V$_1$, on the right side of the sternum between the fourth and fifth intercostal spaces. The negative electrode is placed just below the left midclavicle. Comparably, an MCL$_6$ reading can be obtained by placing the positive electrode at the V$_6$ position. The negative electrode remains below the left clavicle. The unipolar V$_6$ is thus simulated.

Other leads

A modified CR lead (*C* = chest position for positive electrode; *R* = right arm for negative electrode) is often useful to better visualize P waves and to simulate V$_1$. The positive electrode is placed on the right sternal border in the position of V$_1$. The negative electrode is placed under the right clavicle (opposite to that of MCL$_1$).

Ambulatory patients on telemetry can be monitored with both the electrodes at midthorax to minimize artifact. The negative electrode is placed over the manubrium and the positive electrode just above the xiphisternum.

Summary

There are unipolar and bipolar leads. The unipolar leads compare the electrical potentials at particular lead sites with the zero potential at the heart center. The bipolar leads compare the electrical potentials between two lead sites, a negative electrode and a positive electrode.

The cardiac vectors sensed through these leads are recorded according to the magnitude and direction of current flow. This recording is called an ECG.

If a current flows toward a positive electrode, a positive deflection is written. If the current is toward the negative electrode, a negative deflection is written. An equiphasic deflection is the result of the mean vector approaching the axis of a lead at a perpendicular. Knowing the position of the positive electrodes of the leads in the frontal plane, one can then determine the electrical axis of the heart.

CHAPTER 5

Electrical activation of the normal heart

Configuration of the normal ECG

The normal ECG is composed of a P wave, a QRS complex, and a T wave (Fig. 5-1). The P wave represents atrial depolarization and the QRS complex, ventricular depolarization. The T wave reflects the phase of rapid depolarization of the ventricles.

P wave

The duration of the P wave (not over 0.11 sec in the normal person) indicates the time it takes for the depolarization current to pass through the atrial musculature. Because the atria are thin-walled structures, a small de-

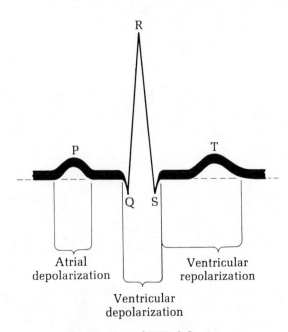

Fig. 5-1. Normal ECG deflections.

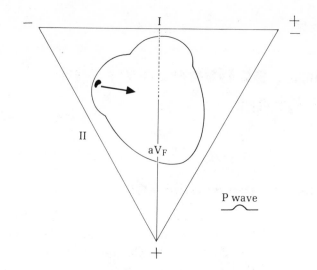

Fig. 5-2. P vector related to the axes of leads I, II, and aV_F.

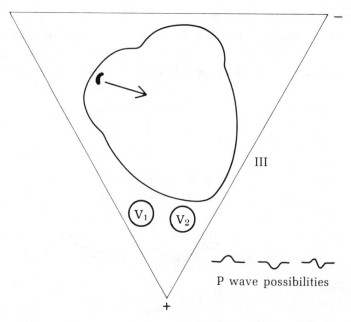

Fig. 5-3. P vector related to the axes of leads *III*, *V₁*, and *V₂*.

flection, not normally more than 3 mm in height, is written. Furthermore, since the P vector is traveling in a leftward and inferior direction, the current flows toward the positive terminals of leads I, II, and aV_F. A positive deflection is therefore written in these leads (Fig. 5-2). Deflections in aV_L and V₃ to V₆ are often positive but may normally be negative or diphasic.

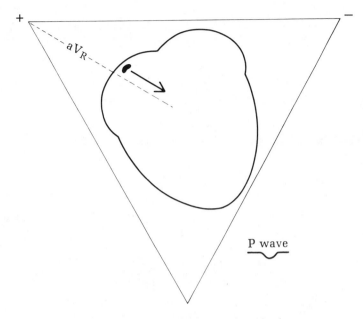

Fig. 5-4. P vector related to the axis of lead aV_R.

Depending on the position of the heart in the body and on the orientation of the atrial vector to the positive terminals, the P wave may be upright, diphasic, flat, or inverted in leads III, V_1, and V_2 (Fig. 5-3). The P wave is usually biphasic in V_1 and V_2 because the activation of the right atrium (anterior vector) and that of the left atrium (posterior vector) are recorded sequentially. The axes of these two leads are anterior-posterior on the horizontal plane.

The P wave is normally inverted in lead aV_R because the vector travels away from this electrode (Fig. 5-4).

Ventricular complex

The shape of the ventricular complex is determined by the orientation of the instant-to-instant vectors to the lead axis.

Fig. 5-5 illustrates the sequence of ventricular depolarization from instant to instant during the cardiac cycle. Vector 1 represents the initial forces, which are normally septal from left to right. An instant later, depolarization will spread to other regions of the ventricles, from endocardium to epicardium. Vectors 2 through 10 are representative of this spread of electrical current, which is repeated consistently, without variation, and at regular intervals in the normal heart.

In Fig. 5-6 the instant-to-instant cardiac vectors are redrawn as though they were all generated from the same point at the center of the heart. If the

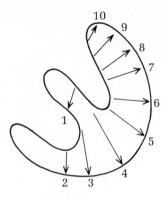

Fig. 5-5. Sequence of electrical activation during the cardiac cycle.

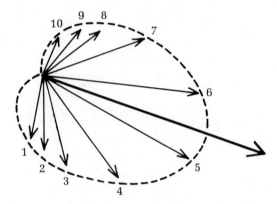

Fig. 5-6. Instant-to-instant cardiac vectors forming the QRS loop. The darker arrow indicates the mean cardiac vector and the axis of the heart.

direction and magnitude of all these vectors are added, the result is the mean vector, indicated by the darker arrow. This is also the axis of the heart. If one wishes to call attention to the sequence in which the instant-to-instant vectors are generated, a line can be drawn from the head of the first arrow around to the last arrow. This is known as the QRS loop.

VENTRICULAR COMPLEX AS SEEN IN THE LIMB LEADS

Figs. 5-7 shows the instant-to-instant electrical events of the heart and how they relate to the axis of the bipolar limb leads. The numbers shown for the ventricular complex correspond to the cardiac vectors. It is noted that a vector which flows toward the negative terminal of the lead inscribes a negative deflection. As the current becomes perpendicular to the lead axis, the deflection returns to the isoelectric (neither negative nor positive) point and then becomes positive when the current swings toward the positive terminal of the lead.

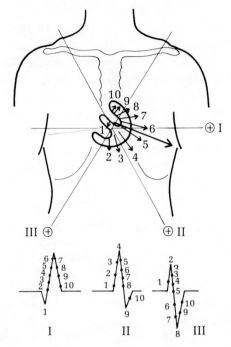

Fig. 5-7. Instant-to-instant cardiac vectors related to the bipolar limb leads. The numbers on the ventricular complexes correspond to the cardiac vectors.

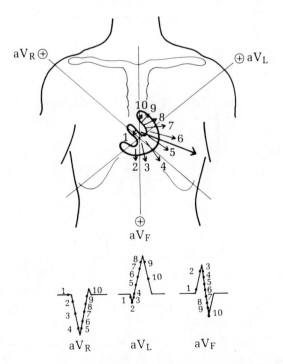

Fig. 5-8. Instant-to-instant cardiac vectors related to the unipolar limb leads. The numbers on the ventricular complexes correspond to the cardiac vectors.

Fig. 5-8 relates the cardiac instant-to-instant vectors to the axes of the unipolar limb leads.

In Figs. 5-7 and 5-8 note the similarities in morphology between the complexes seen in I and aV_L and note only in these two limb leads is septal activation seen as a small negative deflection (q wave). The reasons are that septal activation is a left-right force and the axes of these two leads are also in that direction. In the other limb leads septal activation can be lost in the complex reflecting activation of the walls of the heart. As stated earlier in axis determination, leads I and II should always be positive or at least not more negative than equiphasic. Lead III may be positive or negative and still be normal.

VENTRICULAR ACTIVATION AS SEEN IN THE PRECORDIAL LEADS

Since the axes of the chest leads are on a horizontal plane, it is best to consider a sagittal section of the heart within the chest cage (Fig. 5-9). Vector 1 represents IV septal depolarization, and vectors 2 to 7 represent the sequential activation of the two ventricles—from endocardium to epicardium.

Axis determination is not made with the precordial leads. In fact, the axis of the heart can be shifting back and forth from RAD to LAD, and the precordial leads may show no change at all. These leads do, however, give valuable information about anterior and posterior forces, and because of their proximity to the surface of the heart, precordial leads are helpful in localizing pathological changes in the myocardium. The six positive electrodes of

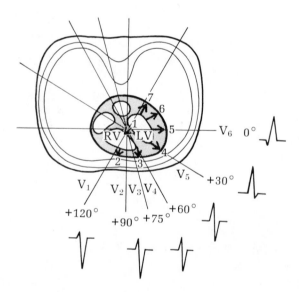

Fig. 5-9. Ventricular activation as seen in the precordial leads.

the precordial leads form a fourth of a circle around the heart, beginning on the right side of the sternum, over the right ventricle, and ending on the left lateral chest wall just over the left ventricle. Remember that the left ventricle is much larger than the right and that left ventricular activation is a leftward, posterior, and inferior force that completely overshadows the electrical activation of the right ventricle. Now look at Fig. 5-9, and you will appreciate why the R waves become taller (R wave progression) and the S waves smaller as the positive electrode moves closer and closer to the left ventricle.

In V_1 the initial little r wave is reflective of both septal and right ventricular forces. However, when right ventricular activation is still just beginning, the dominant leftward force of the left ventricle produces a deep S wave. Thus a narrow rS complex is normal for V_1, although the little r wave may be absent and V_1 still be normal. Electrical activation of the right ventricle is only seen in abnormal circumstances: right bundle branch block, when it is delayed; in some cases of right ventricular hypertrophy, when it dominates; in true posterior myocardial infarction, when posterior forces are lost; and in type B WPW, when right ventricular activation is early.

In V_6 one can detect septal activation very nicely. Because the axis of this lead is from left to right (Fig. 5-9), septal activation is reflected by a small, narrow q wave (as in I and aV_L). Of course this narrow little q wave will be absent when septal activation is abnormal, as in left bundle branch block or anterior septal myocardial infarction.

T wave

The T wave is the result of vectors generated during the repolarization process in the ventricle. At this time the ventricles are in a refractory condition, and a stimulus during the T wave may precipitate a serious ventricular arrhythmia, especially if it occurs during the vulnerable period (from approximately the peak of the T wave to its end).

ELECTROPHYSIOLOGY

Contrary to expectation, the first ventricular area to depolarize (the IV septum) is not the first part to repolarize. If it were, a negative T wave would be inscribed. Rather, the epicardium is the first to repolarize. This is thought to occur because the endocardium recovers more slowly than the epicardium as a result of the pressures of contraction and reduction in coronary blood flow. The repolarization process, then, passes from epicardium to endocardium.

In Fig. 5-10 it can be seen that the depolarization process passes from endocardium to epicardium and that the current is also oriented in this direction (from negative to positive). Although the repolarization process proceeds in the opposite direction (from epicardium to endocardium), the *current still flows from negative to positive*. The vector is therefore oriented toward the positive electrode, causing a positive T wave to be inscribed.

FACTORS CHANGING THE SEQUENCE OF REPOLARIZATION

Anything that changes normal repolarization as described also changes the T wave.

Slow conduction resulting from bundle branch block, ventricular extrasystoles, or ventricular hypertrophy may cause a change in the polarity of the T wave. These conditions change the direction of the depolarization current (mean electrical axis) and thus influence the repolarization process. For example, in left bundle branch block the right ventricle begins to repolarize before the left ventricle, producing a T wave of opposite polarity to that of the QRS.

Prolonged periods of depolarization in portions of the ventricle also change the sequence of repolarization. Ischemia—whether acute, chronic, or associated with coronary occlusion—is the most common cause of increased periods of depolarization. In the presence of ischemia the period of depolarization increases disproportionately.

For example, if there is prolonged depolarization in the apex, the apex will be unable to repolarize first as is normal. The base of the heart therefore repolarizes first, causing a vector in the direction opposite to the normal.

EFFECT OF TOXIC CONDITIONS

Even the slightest change in the period of depolarization of only one portion of the ventricles can cause T wave changes. T wave abnormalities are sensitive indicators of a variety of conditions, including acid-base imbalance,

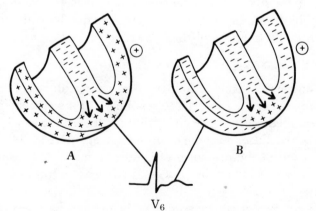

Fig. 5-10. A, Depolarization. **B**, Repolarization.

metabolic diseases, hyperventilation, autonomic hyperactivity, and effects of various drugs.

Definition of QRS deflections

Since the deflections of the ECG are the result of cardiac vectors and their relationship to the axes of the leads, the QRS complex is normally shaped differently in the various leads. The tracing made through each lead represents a view of the heart from another angle.

A baseline may be seen to run the length of the ECG tracing. This is known as the *isoelectric line.* It is present whenever there is no current flowing in the heart; that is, when the heart is either all negative after depolarization or all positive after repolarization.

Fig. 5-11 illustrates how to describe the ventricular complex. A deflection above the line is a positive deflection. A deflection below the line is a negative deflection. All positive deflections are R waves. If there is more than one positive deflection, the second one is called R prime (R′). A negative deflection before the R wave is a Q wave. A negative deflection that occurs after the R wave is an S wave. Sometimes there is no positive deflection at all. The sole negative deflection would be called a QS complex.

The use of lower and upper case letters is a convenient means of signifying the relative sizes of the component waves. The term *QRS* is used collectively.

ECG paper

Time is measured on the horizontal plane. Each small square on the ECG paper is 1 mm in length and represents 0.04 sec in time. The larger square that is defined by the heavier line is 5 mm in length and represents 0.2 sec in time.

Amplitude (voltage) is measured on the vertical plane. All diagnostic twelve-lead ECGs are standardized so that 1 mV is equal to 10 mm (two large squares).

The single vertical lines above the ECG grid are 3 inches apart and represent 3 sec intervals (Fig. 5-12).

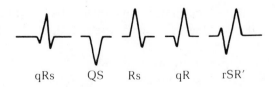

qRs   QS   Rs   qR   rSR′

Fig. 5-11. QRS deflections.

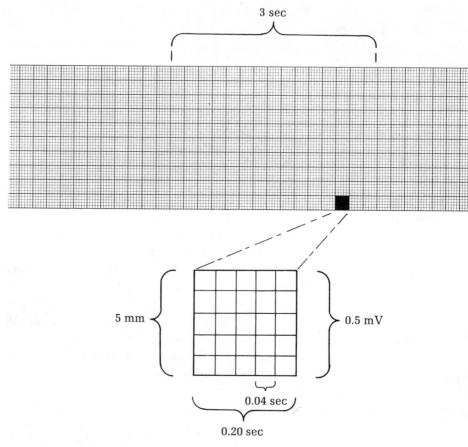

Fig. 5-12. ECG grid.

Calculation of heart rate

ECG tracings may be used to calculate heart rate as follows:
1. Count the number of cycles in a 6-sec strip and multiply by 10. This method can be used when the rhythm is either regular or irregular.
2. Count the number of large squares between two R waves and divide into 300. This method is accurate only if the rhythm is regular.
3. Measure the time interval in seconds between two R waves and divide into 60. For example, if the distance between R waves of two consecutive beats is 0.60 sec, the heart rate is 100. This method is accurate only if the rhythm is regular.
4. For more rapid rhythms or to calculate a rapid atrial rate, count the number of small squares (0.04 sec) between R waves or P waves and divide into 1500. This method is accurate only if the rhythm is regular.

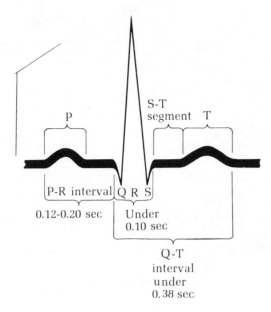

Fig. 5-13. ECG intervals.

Meaning and duration of ECG intervals

The *P-R interval* (Fig. 5-13) is normally between 0.12 and 0.20 sec. It represents the length of time from the beginning of atrial activation to the beginning of ventricular activation. It is measured from the beginning of the P wave to the first ventricular deflection.

The *QRS duration* is normally between 0.06 and 0.10 sec. It represents ventricular conduction time and is measured from the beginning of ventricular activity to its completion, when the tracing returns again to the isoelectric line.

The *Q-T interval* varies with the heart rate. It is measured from the onset of ventricular activity to the end of the T wave. With average heart rates of between 65 and 90/min, the Q-T interval is normally less than half the preceding R-R interval.

Artifacts

An artifact is any product on the ECG that is not caused by the currents generated during the cardiac cycle. Artifacts include alternating current (AC) interference, somatic tremor, wandering baseline, standardization, and external cardiac massage.

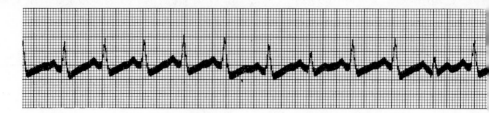

Fig. 5-14. AC interference.

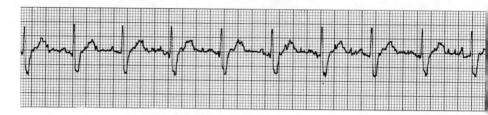

Fig. 5-15. Somatic tremor.

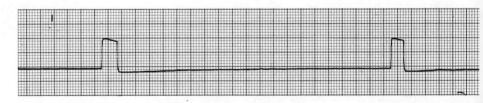

Fig. 5-16. Wandering baseline.

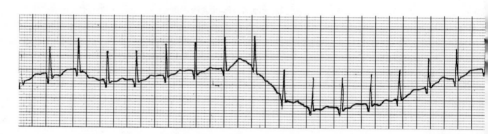

Fig. 5-17. Standardization.

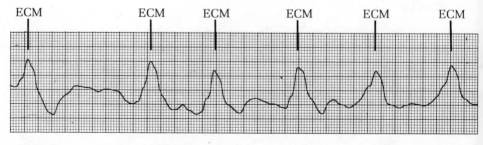

ECM   ECM   ECM   ECM   ECM   ECM

Fig. 5-18. External cardiac massage.

AC INTERFERENCE

AC interference is caused by leakage of the electric power used in the hospital or office. This current pulses or alternates at the rate of 60 cps. A magnifying glass will show exactly sixty even, regular spikes in a 1-sec interval (Fig. 5-14).

SOMATIC TREMOR

Body tremor presents an entirely different picture (Fig. 5-15). There is a grossly uneven, tremulous baseline. It is often seen in patients experiencing tension—the electrical potentials of their "tensed" muscles are picked up by the electrodes.

WANDERING BASELINE

A wandering baseline is an artifact in which the complexes are present but the baseline is undulating (Fig. 5-16).

STANDARDIZATION

An artifact deliberately introduced by the operator so that the interpreter can compare the relationship of the complexes with a known electrical stimulus (Fig. 5-17) is called a standardization artifact. A 1 mV stimulus should cause the stylus to deflect 10 mm (two large squares). If it does not, the operator adjusts the controls until this result is achieved.

EXTERNAL CARDIAC MASSAGE

The complexes sometimes produced by external cardiac massage (ECM) may resemble regular, broad ventricular beats (Fig. 5-18).

Summary

The normal ECG is composed of a P wave, a QRS complex, and a T wave. The morphology of these deflections is dependent on the orientation of the cardiac vector to the lead axis. The deflections are recorded on grid paper that measures time and amplitude (voltage). The strength of the vector, its direction, and its speed are thus measured.

CHAPTER 6

Arrhythmias originating in the sinus node

Normal atrial depolarization

The thin-walled muscle of the atrium produces a weak vector. This is recorded on the ECG as a small P wave, which in some leads may be barely visible. Impulses originating in the sinus node travel the same pathway through the atria each time. Therefore the atrial vector is normally of uniform strength and direction, so that all the P waves in one lead are identical in shape (Fig. 6-1). The normal P wave should probably not be longer than 0.11 sec or more than 3 mm high.

Normally the sinus node depolarizes at regular intervals, between 60 and 100 times/min. An arrhythmia is present (Fig. 6-2) if (1) the rate of depolarization is (a) too fast, (b) too slow, or (c) irregular or (2) the depolarization (a) is too weak to propagate or (b) fails to produce a sufficiently strong stimulus altogether.

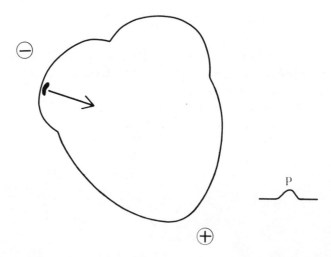

Fig. 6-1. P vector related to a monitoring lead axis and the resultant deflection.

SINUS TACHYCARDIA

In sinus tachycardia the impulses originate regularly, as they should in the sinus node. The current travels along its usual path through the atria and ventricles. The heart rate, however, is faster than normal (100 to 160). The tracing in Fig. 6-3 shows a rate of 140 beats/min. The pacemaker is the sinus node and conduction is normal.

In acute myocardial infarction, sinus tachycardia may be one of the first signs of congestive heart failure, cardiogenic shock, pulmonary embolism, or infarct extension. It is a normal response of the heart to the demand for increased blood flow, occurring with exercise, emotion, pain, fever, or hyperthyroidism. Sinus tachycardia is also caused by drugs such as atropine, quinidine, and adrenaline. There is a differential diagnosis between sinus tachycardia and paroxysmal supraventricular tachycardia. This is discussed on p. 87.

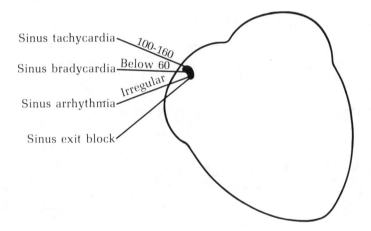

Fig. 6-2. Arrhythmias originating in the sinus node.

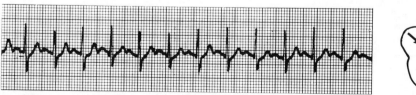

Fig. 6-3. Sinus tachycardia.

SINUS BRADYCARDIA

In sinus bradycardia the pacemaker is the sinus node and conduction is normal. The rhythm is regular, but the rate (below 60 beats/min) is too slow. In the tracing shown in Fig. 6-4 the rate is 38 beats/min.

In acute myocardial infarction, sinus bradycardia may be the result of increased vagal tone and may or may not be accompanied by hypotension. Normally, sinus bradycardia occurs in trained athletes and during sleep.

SINUS ARRHYTHMIA

The pacemaker is the sinus node, and conduction is normal in sinus arrhythmia. However, the rhythm is irregular. Sinus arrhythmia is considered to be present when the difference between the shortest P-P interval and the longest P-P interval is greater than 0.12 sec. These variations in rate are usually due to the vagal effect of respiration on the heart. The rate increases with inspiration and decreases with expiration.

The difference between the two intervals marked in Fig. 6-5 is 0.26 sec. It is a sinus arrhythmia. The rate is normal at 75 beats/min.

SINOATRIAL (SA) BLOCK AND SINUS ARREST

If a P wave does not appear when it is supposed to, this is usually the result of either failure of the sinus impulse to propagate to the atrial tissue (second-degree SA block, type 1 or 2) or failure of the sinus node to generate an

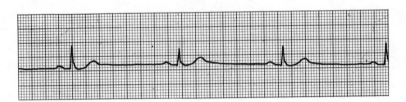

Fig. 6-4. Sinus bradycardia.

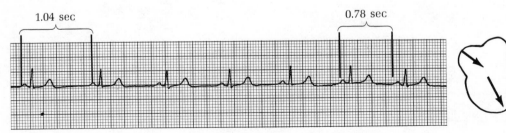

1.04 sec   0.78 sec

Fig. 6-5. Sinus arrhythmia.

impulse at all (sinus arrest). This may occur in normal persons as a result of excessive vagal stimulation. In acute inferior wall myocardial infarction, SA block or sinus arrest may be the result of occlusion of the right coronary artery soon after it leaves its origin in the aorta. It is this artery that supplies the sinus node in 55% of individuals. Other causes include acute myocarditis, digitalis, quinidine, acetylcholine, and potassium.

ECG criteria

Because the activity of the sinus node is not seen on the ECG, it is difficult and sometimes impossible to determine the mechanism involved. Some clues, when present, are helpful and will now be discussed.

SA block. SA block represents a regularly firing sinus node with a disturbance in conduction, which may be either type 1 or 2.

Type 1 (SA Wenckebach) is recognized because of lengthening P-P intervals and pauses that are twice the shortest cycle. The P-R intervals are all the same as long as AV conduction is intact. With each beat there is an increase in the length of time it takes for the sinus impulse to travel from the sinus node to the atrial tissue, until finally a beat is not conducted at all. The greatest increment in conduction time usually occurs between the first and second beats, thus producing a shortening of the P-P intervals before the pause. Fig. 6-6 illustrates type 1 SA block. Note that the P-R intervals are all the same, since the conduction problem in this case is not atrioventricular.

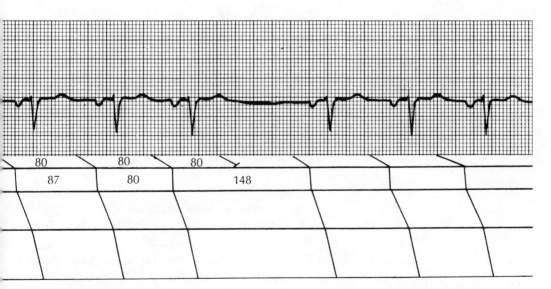

Fig. 6-6. Type 1 SA block, or sinus node Wenckebach. Note the shortening P-P intervals. (From Conover, M. H.: Cardiac arrhythmias; exercises in pattern interpretation, ed. 2, St. Louis, 1978, The C. V. Mosby Co.)

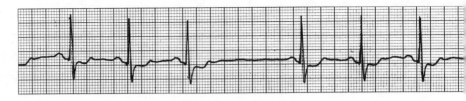

Fig. 6-7. Type 2 SA block. Note that the P-P interval spanning the pause is twice that of the si▮ cycle.

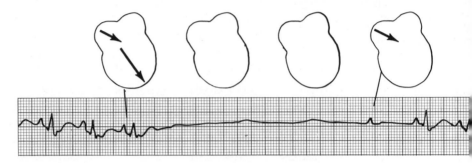

Fig. 6-8. Sinus arrest.

This tracing represents a conduction ratio of 4 : 3; that is, for every four sin▮ discharges, three are conducted to the atrial musculature and produce waves.

Type 2 is recognized because the P-P interval of the pause is just twice th▮ of the basic sinus rhythm. In this arrhythmia a sinus impulse is blocked wit▮ out any increment in conduction time preceding. Fig. 6-7 is a type 2 SA bloc▮ Note that the P-P interval of the pause is twice that of the basic sin▮ rhythm. In the next chapter a far more common arrhythmia that mimics ℂ block, the nonconducted PAC, will be discussed.

Sinus arrest. Sinus arrest represents a marked depression in sinus no▮ automaticity and is diagnosed when the P-P interval of the pause is not multiple of the sinus cycle. Such is the case in Fig. 6-8.

SICK SINUS SYNDROME

The term "sick sinus syndrome" is sometimes used when a patient p▮ sents with cerebral dysfunction secondary to sinus node dysfunction, whi▮ may be either intrinsic or mediated by the autonomic nervous system. Ori▮ inally the term described the sinus arrest following cardioversion for atr▮ fibrillation, but it is now used whenever cerebral perfusion is adversely inf▮ enced by any of the following arrhythmias: severe sinus bradycardia, sin▮ arrest, SA block, sinus bradycardia with recurring atrial fibrillation, a▮ bradycardia-tachycardia syndrome.

ummary

The arrhythmias originating in the sinus node are sinus tachycardia, sinus bradycardia, sinus arrhythmia, SA block, and sinus arrest. In all these arrhythmias the sinus node, as it should be, is the pacemaker of the heart. However, its rate is either too fast, too slow, irregular, or inconsistent.

ferences

Goldberger, E.: Treatment of cardiac emergencies, ed. 2, St. Louis, 1977, The C. V. Mosby Co.

Watanabe, Y., and Dreifus, L. S.: Cardiac arrhythmias; electrophysiologic basis for clinical interpretation, New York, 1977, Grune & Stratton, Inc.

3. Marriott, H. J. L.: Practical electrocardiography, ed. 6, Baltimore, 1977, The Williams & Wilkins Co.

CHAPTER 7

Supraventricular ectopics

The term *supraventricular* refers to the area above the bifurcation of th
bundle of His. An ectopic complex or rhythm is a single complex or a su
tained rhythm originating from a focus other than the sinus node. Supr:
ventricular ectopics are, then, complexes or rhythms originating outside th
sinus node but not below the bifurcation of the bundle of His. This holds tru
even though the bundle of His penetrates into the ventricular septum.

In this chapter all supraventricular ectopics (atrial, junctional, and A
nodal reentry) are grouped together to clarify mechanisms, define clinic:
implications, and resolve confusion surrounding terminology (Fig. 7-1

Some supraventricular ectopics originate in the atria due to enhance
automaticity; others originate in the AV junction for the same reason an
may at times produce AV dissociation.

Still other supraventricular ectopics originate in the atria or the AV jun
tion due to enhanced automaticity but are sustained by an AV nodal reentr
circuit rather than continued rapid firing of that single focus (p. 27).

Furthermore, supraventricular ectopics may be either premature or e

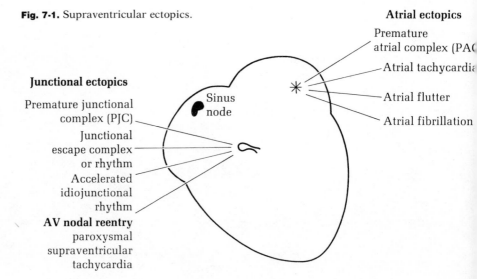

Fig. 7-1. Supraventricular ectopics.

Atrial ectopics

Premature
atrial complex (PA(

Atrial tachycardi:

Atrial flutter

Atrial fibrillation

Junctional ectopics

Premature junctional
complex (PJC)

Junctional
escape complex
or rhythm

Accelerated
idiojunctional
rhythm

AV nodal reentry
paroxysmal
supraventricular
tachycardia

Sinus
node

cape. Thus the complex itself may be the same but the etiology and clinical implications completely different.

In order to illustrate these similarities and differences more clearly, the discussion in this chapter will be according to the following classification.

Atrial ectopic mechanisms
    Premature atrial complex (PAC)—enhanced automaticity
    Atrial tachycardia *(usually with AV block)*—enhanced automaticity or intra-atrial
        reentry
    Chaotic atrial tachycardia—enhanced automaticity (multifocal)
    Atrial flutter—mechanism uncertain, probably intra-atrial reentry
    Atrial fibrillation—often initiated by a single PAC
    Atrial escape complex—normal atrial mechanism
Junctional ectopic mechanisms
    Premature junctional complex (PJC)—enhanced automaticity
    Accelerated idiojunctional rhythm—enhanced automaticity at a rate of less
        than 100 beats/min but greater than the inherent rate of the AV junction (40 to
        60 beats/min); often results in AV dissociation*
    Junctional tachycardia—enhanced automaticity at a rate over 100 beats/min
        (usually does not exceed 130 beats/min)
    Junctional escape complexes—normal junctional mechanism
    Junctional escape rhythms—normal junctional mechanism; often results in AV
        dissociation*
AV nodal reentry mechanism
    Paroxysmal supraventricular tachycardia (AV nodal reciprocating tachycardia)—
        may begin with a single PAC or PJC but is sustained by AV nodal reentry

Atrial ectopic mechanisms
PREMATURE ATRIAL COMPLEX (PAC)
P′ wave

When the atrial impulse originates at a point other than the sinus node, the resultant deflection is called a P′ wave. The ectopic focus may be anywhere in the atria. The shape of the P′ wave depends on the orientation of the vector to the axis of the lead. If the ectopic focus is in the vicinity of the sinus node, the resultant P′ wave closely resembles the normal sinus P wave. Its sole distinguishing feature may be that it is premature. However, if the ectopic focus is located so that its vector takes a different path, the resultant P′ wave has a different shape from that of the normal P wave.

In the setting of the coronary care unit atrial premature beats may warn of electrolyte imbalance, hypoxia, digitalis toxicity, or onset of congestive heart failure. Their appearance should elicit a physical assessment and clinical evaluation of the patient.

---

*AV dissociation is not discussed in this book under a separate heading, since it is merely a symptom of other problems. It will be illustrated and explained under the arrhythmias that produce it.

Fig. 7-2 depicts sinus bradycardia with a rate of 48. Mark off the first tw normal sinus P waves. Bring this mark across the strip, and you will eas find the premature atrial complex. It occurs early, before the expected sin P wave. It is also shaped differently, being a little narrower and more point than the normal sinus P waves.

The PACs in Fig. 7-3 are hidden in the preceding T waves. Ectopic P wav (P') commonly hide in T waves. Whenever there is an irregularity, it is we to closely examine and compare the T waves. They should all be the sar shape. In Fig. 7-3 there are two T waves that are more pointed and peake than the others. They have been distorted by P' waves and are followed by normal ventricular response.

Bigeminal PACs

In Fig. 7-4 every other P wave is ectopic. Each P' wave is followed by normal ventricular response.

Nonconducted PACs

Now mark off the first two normal sinus P waves shown in Fig. 7-5 on separate piece of paper. Bring these marks across the strip. At the point which the rhythm becomes irregular, a P' wave can be seen on the T wav You may think this is only a T wave until you carefully examine and con pare it with the T waves following the other complexes. You will find tha they are flatter and not as pointed. The ventricular response to this ectop P wave is absent. Conduction is blocked because of a physiological refract riness in the ventricles. The PAC occurs before the ventricles are ready to ac cept it. Therefore this atrial stimulus is not conducted.

Nonconducted PACs are commonly the cause of unexpected pauses an therefore should be suspected before SA block or sinus arrest is considere

Bigeminal nonconducted PACs

Bigeminal nonconducted PACs can very closely simulate sinus bradyca dia. This mechanism should be suspected when the bradycardia is of sudde onset. In Fig. 7-6 bigeminal nonconducted PACs exactly simulate abrupt pro found sinus bradycardia. The first P' wave (in the third T wave) is conducte normally. The bigeminal rhythm then continues with a P' wave in every wave. It is helpful to note that the P' wave is not part of the electrophys iology of the T wave. Therefore, if P' waves occur at the same time as the waves, they will distort the T wave differently each time. Note in Fig. 7-6 tha not only are the T waves before the pauses different from the normal T waves they are also different from each other.

Fig. 7-7 depicts a sinus tachycardia with two nonconducted PACs. If th bigeminal pattern had been sustained, a diagnosis of sinus bradycardi

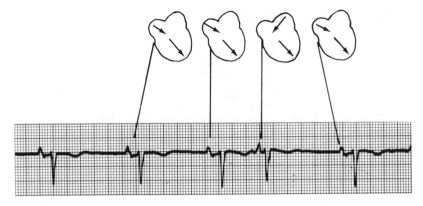

Fig. 7-2. Single premature atrial complex (PAC).

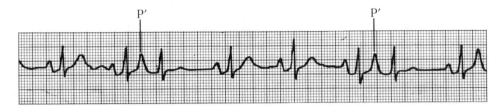

Fig. 7-3. PACs hidden in the T waves.

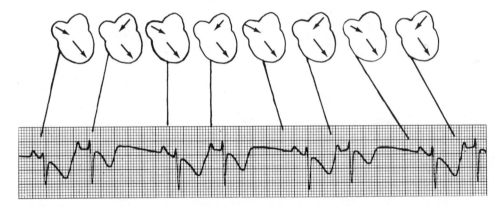

Fig. 7-4. Bigeminal PACs.

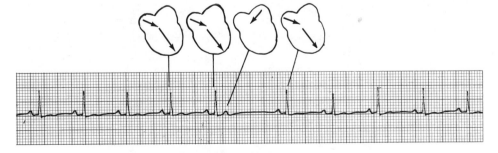

Fig. 7-5. Nonconducted PAC.

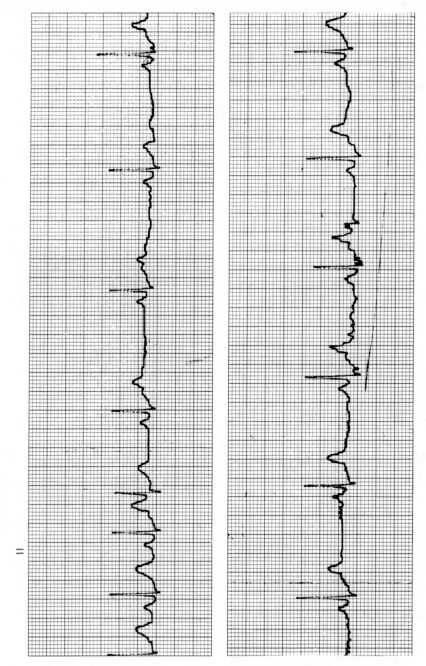

Fig. 7-6. Bigeminal nonconducted PACs simulating abrupt, profound sinus bradycardia (continuous tracings). (From Conover, M. H.: Cardiac arrhythmias: exercises in pattern interpretation, ed. 2, St. Louis, 1978, The C. V. Mosby Co.)

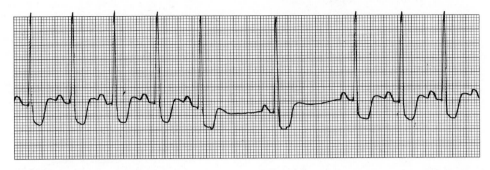

Fig. 7-7. Sinus tachycardia with two nonconducted PACs. Notice the irregular shape of the two T waves preceding the pauses.

II

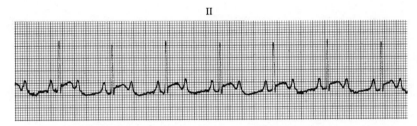

Fig. 7-8. Atrial tachycardia with 2:1 AV conduction.

would perhaps have been made. Note the irregular shape of T waves preceding the pauses.

ATRIAL TACHYCARDIA

In atrial tachycardia the atria are stimulated at a rate of 150 to 250 beats/ min. This may either result from the rapid firing of an area of enhanced automaticity within the atria or an intra-atrial reentry mechanism utilizing a pathway through the sinus node or internodal pathways. The AV node normally protects the ventricles from rapid ectopic atrial rhythms. Therefore atrial tachycardia is usually accompanied by AV block.

In Fig. 7-8 two P' waves can be seen from every QRS complex. Mark off two consecutive P' waves. Bring this interval along the tracing and you will find that the P' waves occur at regular intervals. The atrial rate is 132. The ventricular rate is 66. This is probably atrial tachycardia with "block."

In order to differentiate this arrhythmia from sinus tachycardia with second-degree block, one would need to see the onset of the tachycardia and to compare the morphology of the P waves. It is helpful to remember that both the sinus node and the AV node are under the control of the vagus nerve so that when the sinus node speeds up, so does AV conduction. Thus a sinus tachycardia of 132 would conduct every beat (given an intact AV conduction

V₁

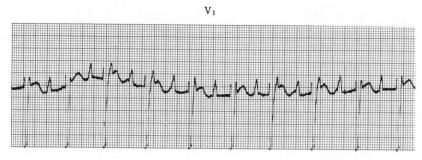

Fig. 7-9. Atrial tachycardia with 2:1 AV conduction.

path), whereas an ectopic atrial focus firing at that rate would more than likely be blocked.

Fig. 7-9 illustrates another atrial tachycardia with block. One P′ wave is partially hidden by the QRS complex. The downward slope of it can just be seen at the end of the rS complex, making it appear to be an rSR′. The atrial rate is 180, and the ventricular rate is 90.

CHAOTIC ATRIAL TACHYCARDIA

In Fig. 7-10 at least five different P′ waves can be seen. This is indicative of multifocal atrial ectopics and is sometimes termed *chaotic atrial tachycardia*. It is an arrhythmia commonly seen in patients with chronic lung conditions.

ATRIAL FLUTTER

Atrial flutter is usually initiated by a PAC and is thought to be supported by an intra-atrial reentry pathway. In this case there are P′ waves at a rate somewhere between 300 and 350. The atria have been known to respond in a unified fashion even to a rate of 400 or more.

Atrial flutter with block

Here again, as with atrial tachycardia due to enhanced automaticity, the ventricles are protected from the rapid atrial rates of atrial flutter by the refractory state of the AV junction.

The tracing in Fig. 7-11 is an example of atrial flutter with 4:1 AV conduction (block). The atrial rate is 325 beats/min, and the characteristic undulating, sawtooth pattern may be observed. There is a response to every fourth P′ wave; thus the ventricular rate is 80.

Fig. 7-12 illustrates one of the most commonly misdiagnosed arrhythmias, often missed by both the novice and experienced personnel. It is atrial

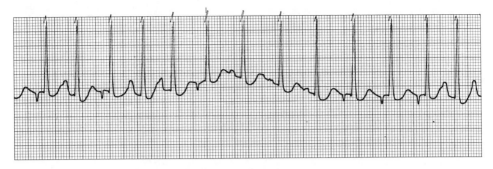

Fig. 7-10. Chaotic atrial tachycardia.

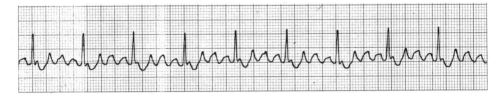

Fig. 7-11. Atrial flutter with 4 : 1 AV conduction.

II

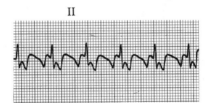

Fig. 7-12. Atrial flutter with 2 : 1 AV conduction.

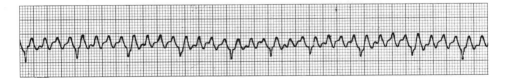

Fig. 7-13. Atrial flutter with variable block.

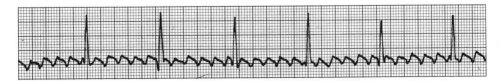

Fig. 7-14. Atrial flutter with AV dissociation.

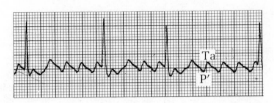

Fig. 7-15. Morphology of *P'* and *Ta* wave in atrial flutter.

flutter with 2:1 block. This is missed because the QRS-T obliterates one of the flutter waves. There are two rules that will help avoid this diagnostic pitfall: (1) whenever the ventricular rate is around 150 beats/min, be suspicious of a hidden P' wave (atrial flutter is commonly 300 beats/min) and (2) in atrial flutter there is commonly a hump going into the QRS complex, which is the repolarization wave of the ectopic atrial beat.

Atrial flutter with variable block

In Fig. 7-13 the ventricles are irregular in their response to a rapid (350 beats/min) atrial stimulus. Responses of 2:1, 3:1, and 4:1 can be seen in this tracing.

Atrial flutter with AV dissociation

When the block at the AV node exceeds 4:1, there may be a pathological cause rather than a functional refractoriness.

In Fig. 7-14 the atrial rate is 300, and the ventricles are beating regularly at a rate of 55. No constant relationship is found between the QRS and the preceding flutter wave, indicating that the ventricles are beating independently.

Morphology of the flutter wave

In atrial flutter the atrial repolarization wave (Ta wave) is clearly seen. In the normal sinus rhythm it is hidden in the QRS complex.

The P' wave is usually the negative deflection of the sawtooth pattern. The Ta wave is the positive deflection (Fig. 7-15).

In atrial flutter the atria beat rapidly and regularly. Therefore a QRS complex may occur at the same time as a P' (flutter) wave. In order to determine the degree of block, it is important to mark off the two or three visible P' waves. When these marks are brought along the tracing, a P' wave is found hidden within the QRS complex.

ATRIAL FIBRILLATION

The atria can respond in an organized fashion to as many as 350 impulses/min and sometimes as many as 400 or more. With a more rapid stim-

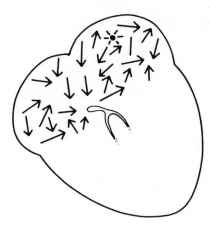

Fig. 7-16. Disorganized electrical activity of atrial fibrillation.

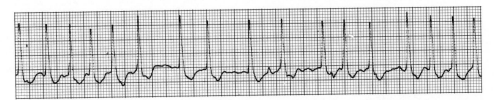

Fig. 7-17. Atrial fibrillation with an uncontrolled ventricular response. Note fine fibrillatory line.

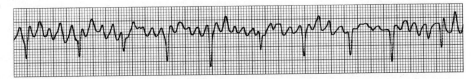

Fig. 7-18. Atrial fibrillation with a controlled ventricular response and a coarse fibrillatory line.

ulus the atrial muscle cells cannot all repolarize in time for the next stimulus. As a result, the ectopic vector is rejected by the refractory cells, and electrical chaos results. Depolarization and repolarization occur, but there is no unified electrical activity. Rather, there are vectors in different directions at different times (Fig. 7-16).

Fibrillatory line

The erratic electrical activity in the atria is reflected on the ECG by a fibrillatory line that may be very fine, as seen in Fig. 7-17; very coarse, as seen in Fig. 7-18; or somewhere in between these two.

When the fibrillatory line is coarse, as in Fig. 7-18, you may at times see what looks like a P wave. Keep in mind the fact that true P waves are regular, all of the same configuration, and usually occur at the same place before each QRS complex.

Atrial fibrillation and AV conduction

Thus far we have established that in atrial fibrillation the P waves are absent and that the disorganized atrial electrical activity is reflected by a wavy fibrillatory line with no set pattern.

Normally the AV node is depolarized regularly by an impulse arriving from the sinus node. In atrial fibrillation there are many vectors (depolarization waves or currents) bombarding the AV node. Some of the action potentials stimulating the AV node are weak. They are therefore not propagated into the ventricles, although they do partially depolarize the AV junction, leaving it refractory to another stimulus (concealed conduction). Thus the ventricular response in atrial fibrillation is irregular.

The ventricular response shown in the tracing of atrial fibrillation in Fig. 7-17 is approximately 140/beats min. In Fig. 7-18 the ventricular rate is approximately 90 beats/min.

Digitalis toxicity in atrial fibrillation will be discussed in the Chapter 9.

ATRIAL ESCAPE COMPLEX (WANDERING PACEMAKER)

Wandering pacemaker is a passive rather than an active arrhythmia and refers to atrial escape as opposed to atrial prematurity. It is sometimes referred to as a shifting pacemaker and is characterized by a P-P' interval that is longer than the normal P-P interval.

In Fig. 7-19 the pacemaker shift is easily seen as the P wave deflection changes from positive to negative. The P-P' interval is 0.09 sec longer than the P-P interval. The ectopic pacemaker is therefore not active and premature (PAC) but is late and passive. The first P' wave is biphasic, indicating either a third ectopic pacemaker somewhere between the sinus and AV nodes or an atrial fusion beat (a collision of sinus and nodal vectors).

Pacemaker shifts may be caused by almost identical intrinsic rates in both nodes. Thus if the sinus node slows down, the AV junction or another focus may depolarize first.

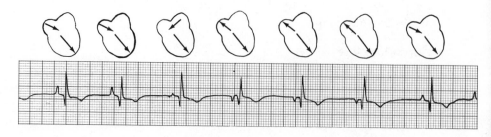

Fig. 7-19. Multifocal atrial escape beats (wandering pacemaker).

Junctional ectopic mechanisms
HISTORICAL BACKGROUND

In 1913 Zahn described what he called "upper-," "mid-," and "low-nodal" rhythms. His descriptive terminology was based on what was thought to be the level of the ectopic pacemaker in the AV node. This conclusion was made because of the shape of the P' wave (inverted in leads II, III, and aV$_F$) and its relation to the QRS complex. If the inverted P' wave immediately preceded the QRS and if a P'-R interval of less than 0.12 sec was present, the focus was said to be in the upper region of the AV node. If the P' wave was buried in the QRS, the focus was said to be centrally located within the AV node. An inverted P' wave immediately following the QRS was said to originate from a focus in the lower region of the AV node.

Today it is known that the configuration of the P wave and its relation to the ventricular complex depend on many factors. The site of impulse formation is certainly one factor that influences on the shape of the P wave. However, anatomical origins of impulse formation from the AV nodal area cannot be determined precisely from the ECG. Furthermore, P-QRS relationships are determined not only by the site of impulse formation but also by the relative speed of anterograde (forward) and retrograde (backward) conduction as well. We will therefore use the broader term, *AV junctional*, to refer to ectopic beats or rhythms that are thought to have originated in this area.

MORPHOLOGY OF JUNCTIONAL BEATS

If the AV junctional region paces the heart, the P' vector must travel in a retrograde direction in order to activate the atria. In leads II, III, and aV$_F$ this current flows away from the positive terminal of the leads and causes a negative P' wave to be recorded (Fig. 7-20).

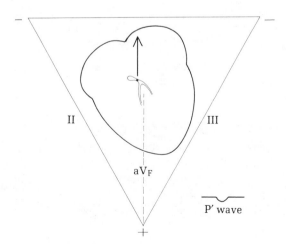

Fig. 7-20. Retrograde activation of the atria and the P' wave in leads II, III, and aV$_F$.

The QRS complex produced by a junctional beat is usually narrow in the absence of intraventricular conduction defects because the impulse arises above the branching portion of the bundle of His and is simultaneously distributed to both ventricles. Of course, with a coexisting intraventricular conduction defect, the QRS is altered.

PREMATURE JUNCTIONAL COMPLEX (PJC)

The three types of junctional premature complexes are illustrated in Fig. 7-21. In *A* the negative P' wave can be seen immediately preceding the third QRS, indicating that retrograde atrial activation preceded anterograde ventricular activation. Note that the P'-R interval is less than 0.12 sec.

In Fig. 7-21, *B*, the P' wave is not seen at all, indicating one of two causes. Either (1) retrograde activation of the atria occurred at the same time as anterograde activation of the ventricles, and thus the P' wave is hidden in the QRS, or (2) retrograde conduction to the atria was blocked, and there is atrial standstill.

In Fig. 7-21, *C*, the P' wave can be seen immediately following the third QRS complex, which is premature. It distorts the S-T segment of that beat. In this case retrograde activation of the atria followed anterograde activation of the ventricles.

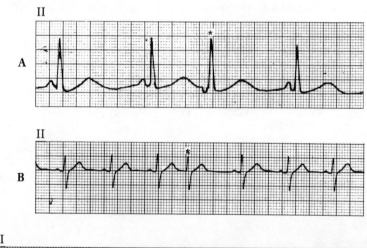

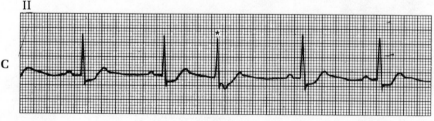

Fig. 7-21. Junctional premature beats.

Where the P' wave occurs relative to the QRS complex is a function of the relative speeds of anterograde and retrograde conduction, plus the location of the ectopic focus.

The main ECG diagnostic criteria for the PJC are that (1) it is premature, (2) the QRS complex is identical in morphology to the sinus-conducted ventricular complexes, and (3) if the P' wave precedes the QRS, it does so by no more than 0.11 sec.

Premature junctional complexes are commonly a manifestation of digitalis toxicity and are the result of enhanced automaticity.

ACCELERATED IDIOJUNCTIONAL RHYTHM

The *accelerated idiojunctional rhythm* occurs because of enhanced automaticity within the AV junction, commonly due to digitalis excess. Its rate is between 62 and 100 beats/min—not a tachycardia in the strict sense of the word but certainly too fast for junctional pacemaker cells. This arrhythmia does not begin abruptly, as does the paroxysmal supraventricular tachycardia. On the contrary, its beginning is insidious. Initially it may manifest itself with a few isolated PJCs. As the rate of the junctional ectopic focus increases to a little more than that of the sinus node, there may be AV dissociation: that is, the junctional focus paces the ventricles while the sinus node paces the atria. Fig. 7-22 shows just such an arrhythmia. Note that the first three beats are sinus conducted but that the fourth beat is a junctional beat that is ever so slightly premature. For the next thirteen complexes this junctional focus retains command of the ventricles while the sinus node paces the atria. As the junctional complexes get more and more premature, the effect is given of P waves *walking into* R waves. Toward the end of the tracing the rate of the sinus node increases enough so that its impulse can once more capture the ventricles.

Whether or not the P wave walks into the R wave is not the important observation. The rate of the junctional ectopic focus is clinically very significant. It should not exceed 60 beats/min. Rates in excess of this value commonly indicate digitalis toxicity. The rate of the junctional focus in Fig. 7-22 is 70 beats/min, an accelerated idiojunctional rhythm. Hemodynamically, as the P wave coincides with the QRS complex, the patient loses the atrial contribution to cardiac output, which may or may not be well tolerated.

Fig. 7-23 illustrates another accelerated idiojunctional rhythm with a rate of 74 beats/min. At the beginning of the tracing the sinus P waves can be seen as a small hump just before, and actually seeming to be a part of, the QRS complex. Toward the middle of the tracing the sinus P waves can be seen behind the QRS. As the sinus rate speeds up to exceed that of the junction, the P waves move to the front of the QRS and finally capture the ventricles toward the end of the tracing.

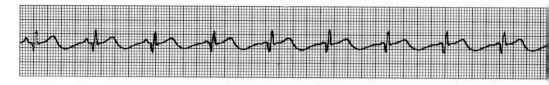

Fig. 7-22. Accelerated idiojunctional rhythm (70 beats/min) with AV dissociation

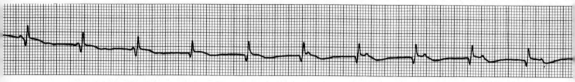

Fig. 7-23. Accelerated idiojunctional rhythm (74 beats/min) with AV dissociation

JUNCTIONAL TACHYCARDIA

When the rate of the accelerated idioventricular focus exceeds 100 beats/ min, it is called *junctional tachycardia*. Fig. 7-24 is such an arrhythmia. The junctional rate is 120 beats/min, and the junctional focus completely dominates both the atria and the ventricles. The negative P' wave can be seen distorting the inverted T wave. It is readily seen if the tracing is turned upside down.

JUNCTIONAL ESCAPE COMPLEXES

Junctional escape occurs when there is undue delay in the arrival of the impulse from the prevailing rhythm. Junctional cells have an inherent rate of 40 to 60 beats/min. Therefore, when the pause in the ECG is long enough, the cells in the AV junction reach threshold and discharge themselves. They are often seen following the pauses created by nonconducted PACs, in type I second-degree heart block, and in sinus bradycardia.

In Fig. 7-25 a junctional escape complex follows a pause created by a nonconducted PAC. The P' wave can be seen distorting the T wave preceding the pause. The QRS following the pause is a junctional escape complex. The sinus P wave preceding it is too close to have conducted.

The clinical implications of junctional escape complexes are completely different from those of junctional premature complexes. The junctional escape is a normal mechanism. In such a case one concentrates on why the pause occurred rather than why the junction escaped, whereas the premature junctional complex is a manifestation of "irritation" in the junction, which should be clinically analyzed.

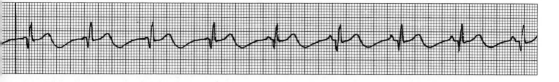

tinuous strips).

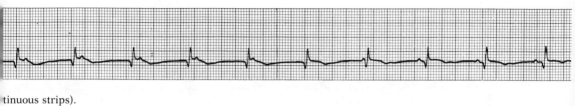

tinuous strips).

Lead II

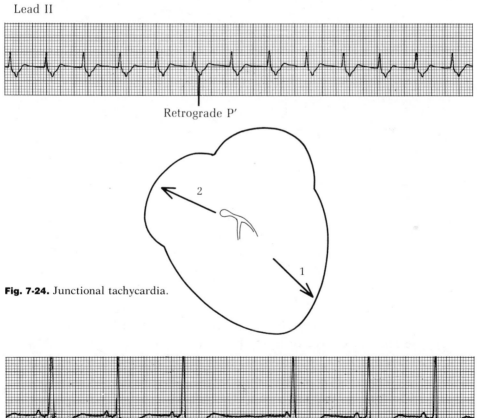

Retrograde P′

Fig. 7-24. Junctional tachycardia.

Fig. 7-25. Junctional escape following a nonconducted PAC.

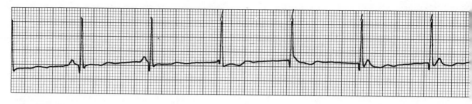

Fig. 7-26. Sinus bradycardia with an appropriate junctional escape rhythm of 58 beats/min, as

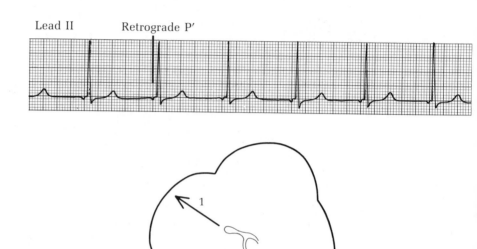

Fig. 7-27. Junctional escape rhythm (60 beats/min). Atrial activation precedes ventricular activation.

JUNCTIONAL ESCAPE RHYTHMS

Junctional escape rhythms normally protect the heart whenever the sinus rhythm is too slow or in the presence of complete AV heart block. At times this arrhythmia may be accompanied by AV dissociation, which implies that AV conduction is intact but the sinus node is beating slower than the normal inherent rate of the junction. Such is the case in Fig. 7-26. When the sinus node slows from a rate of 58 to 55 beats/min, the junction assumes control at its own intrinsic rate of 58. The sinus P waves get closer and closer to the QRS until they enter it and emerge on the other side (walking

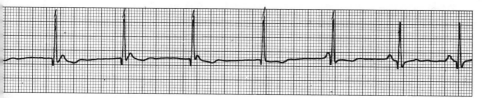

well as AV dissociation (continuous strips).

Lead II

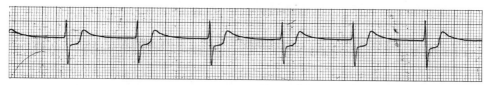

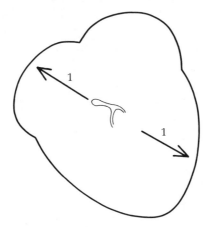

Fig. 7-28. Junctional escape rhythm (57 beats/min). Atrial and ventricular activations occur simultaneously or are blocked.

through). The two pacemakers (sinus and junctional) then beat at approximately the same rate (isorhythmic) until the sinus node accelerates to a rate of 67 and thus regains control of the ventricles (capture).

Fig. 7-27 illustrates a junctional escape rhythm of 60 beats/min that completely dominates both atria and ventricles. The retrograde P′ wave can be seen immediately preceding the QRS complex.

Fig. 7-28 is another junctional escape rhythm of 57 beats/min. P waves are not seen at all in this tracing. They may either be hidden within the QRS complex or not be there due to retrograde block or atrial paralysis.

AV nodal reentry mechanism (paroxysmal supraventricular tachycardia)

Paroxysmal supraventricular tachycardia, or AV nodal reciprocating tachycardia, begins abruptly and ends abruptly. It is usually initiated by a premature atrial or junctional beat and is supported by a reentry circuit through the AV junction. The ventricular rate is usually between 180 and 220 beats/min but may be as slow as 100 or as fast as 250 beats/min. This arrhythmia may often be terminated by vagal maneuvers, is generally self-limiting, and is well tolerated by the healthy heart. This mechanism has been discussed and illustrated on pp. 26 to 27 in Chapter 3. Figs. 7-29 and 7-30 are examples of paroxysmal supraventricular tachycardias that are initiated by PACs. In Fig. 7-29 the P' wave is in the T wave immediately after the fifth QRS. In Fig. 7-30 the P' wave is in the T wave of the fourth QRS.

DIFFERENTIAL DIAGNOSIS AMONG MECHANISMS OF PAROXYSMAL SUPRAVENTRICULAR TACHYCARDIA

Recently Wu et al.[1] and Wellens[2] have published criteria helpful in the ECG determination of the mechanism of paroxysmal supraventricular tachycardia. Fig. 7-31 illustrates these findings.

According to Wu et al., when the mechanism of the tachycardia is AV nodal reentry, the retrograde P' wave is hidden in the QRS 66% of the time because (1) anterograde conduction is usually through the slow pathway and retrograde conduction through the fast pathway and (2) the relationship of

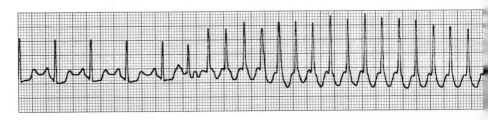

Fig. 7-29. Paroxysmal supraventricular tachycardia. Note the P' wave in the fifth T. A reciprocating tachycardia follows.

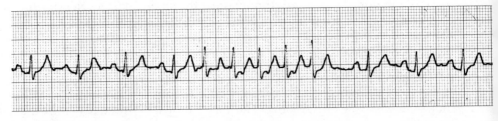

Fig. 7-30. Paroxysmal supraventricular tachycardia. Note the P' wave in the fourth T.

these conduction times results in simultaneous atrial and ventricular activation. The P′ wave follows the QRS when retrograde conduction is slower than usual (30% of the time). Rarely, the P′ wave precedes the QRS, reflective of an anterograde fast pathway and retrograde slow pathway.

When the paroxysmal supraventricular tachycardia is due to a concealed accessory pathway conducting retrogradely (p. 163), the P′ wave always follows the QRS because atrial activation will occur in sequence after the ventricles, that is, ventricles → accessory pathway → atria → AV junction → ventricles, and so on.

When the paroxysmal supraventricular tachycardia is due to sinus or atrial reentry, the P waves usually occur in front of the QRS because atrial rates are slow and AV conduction is not depressed.

DIFFERENTIAL DIAGNOSIS BETWEEN PSVT AND SINUS TACHYCARDIA

1. PSVT begins abruptly with a single PAC or PJC, whereas sinus tachycardia moves slowly into a tachycardia in response to physiological needs.
2. PSVT usually has a rate in excess of 160 beats/min, sometimes reaching as high as 250 when the mechanism is AV nodal reentry, whereas sinus tachycardia usually does not exceed 150 beats/min.
3. PSVT may be abruptly terminated by a vagal maneuver, whereas sinus tachycardia only momentarily slows down.
4. The P wave morphology in PSVT differs from that of the normal sinus P wave in most cases.

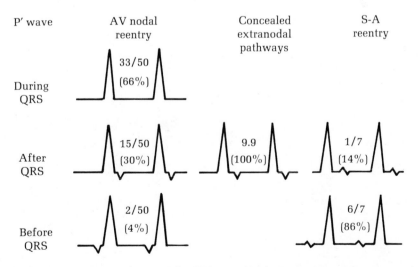

Fig. 7-31. Timing of P waves relative to the QRS complex during paroxysmal supraventricular tachycardia in three groups of patients. (From Wu, D., et al.: Am. J. Cardiol. **41:**1045, 1978.)

Summary

Supraventricular ectopic complexes and rhythms originate outside the normal pacemaker and sinus node and above the bifurcation of the bundle of His. They may be either abnormal premature mechanisms or normal escape mechanisms in response to an abnormality in the sinus node.

The two most common mechanisms involved in these arrhythmias are enhanced automaticity and reentry, either intra-atrial or AV nodal. A third mechanism involving the slow calcium channel is under investigation (pp 29 to 30).

Enhanced automaticity may cause single premature atrial or junctional complexes, atrial tachycardia (usually with AV block), accelerated idiojunctional rhythm (rate 61 to 100 beats/min), or junctional tachycardia (rate over 100 beats/min). Such mechanisms are commonly the result of digitalis excess, acute myocardial infarction, or acute rheumatic fever.

An AV nodal reentry mechanism may be activated by a single premature atrial, junctional, or ventricular premature complex to produce paroxysmal supraventricular tachycardia.

Intra-atrial or sinus reentry mechanisms may be precipitated by a single premature atrial complex.

References

1. Wu, D., et al.: Clinical, electrocardiographic and electrophysiologic observations in patients with paroxysmal supraventricular tachycardia, Am. J. Cardiol. **41:**1045, 1978.

2. Wellens, H. J. J.: Value and limitations of programmed electrical stimulation of the heart in the study and treatment of tachycardias, Circulation **57:**845, 1978.

CHAPTER 8

Ventricular ectopics

A ventricular ectopic is a complex or rhythm that originates in the ventricles (below the branching portion of the bundle of His). Although ventricular ectopics may occur in apparently normal hearts, in the setting of the coronary care unit they may be life threatening. Therefore it is important that they be recognized and treated promptly. It is generally agreed that ventricular ectopy is the result of either reentry or enhanced automaticity in the ventricular conductive system. Recently, triggered activity as a result of afterpotentials has been named as a possible cause of some atrial and ventricular ectopics. These mechanisms have already been discussed in Chapter 3. Ventricular ectopy may be secondary to myocardial ischemia or infarction, hypoxia, drugs, catecholamines, metabolic imbalance, emotional tension, cardiac disease, and a variety of other factors.

Ventricular ectopy may take the form of a premature ventricular complex (PVC), ventricular tachycardia (VT), ventricular fibrillation (VF), accelerated idioventricular rhythm (rate < 100 beats/min), parasystolic rhythm, or ventricular escape.

Premature ventricular complexes (PVCs)

A PVC is recognized because it is broad (>0.11 sec), premature, has an increased amplitude with a T wave of opposite polarity, and has no related P wave. The PVC also almost always has a full compensatory pause, but there are limitations to the value of this pause as proof of ventricular ectopy.

DEPOLARIZATION FOLLOWING A VENTRICULAR ECTOPIC STIMULUS

An ectopic focus stimulating the ventricles is usually located within the His-Purkinje system. The ventricular vector begins at the site of the focus and travels toward the rest of the ventricular muscle mass. The orientation of this vector to the axes of the leads is abnormal, causing an abnormal and different deflection. Because the impulse cannot travel on its usual accelerated path by way of the bundle of His and bundle branches, conduction is delayed, causing a characteristically broad complex.

The shape of a ventricular extrasystole is dependent on the location of the

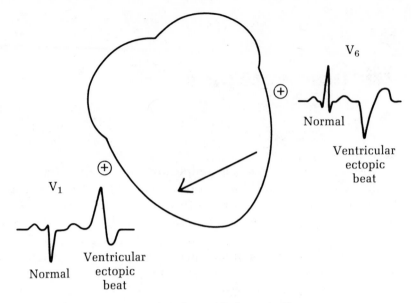

Fig. 8-1. Ectopic ventricular activation.

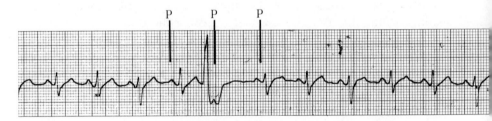

Fig. 8-2. Full compensatory pause. Note that all sinus P waves can be seen.

ectopic focus in the ventricles and on the orientation of the vector to the axis of the lead (Fig. 8-1).

Prematurity

An ectopic focus must depolarize the ventricle before the normal sinus stimulus arrives, or it will itself be depolarized by the normal impulse. The active ventricular extrasystole is therefore always premature, that is, before the next expected ventricular complex.

Full compensatory pause

When a PVC occurs, the atrium is sometimes not affected. The sinus node continues to beat regularly. The P waves therefore occur on time in spite of the ventricular irregularity. There is no ventricular response to the P wave

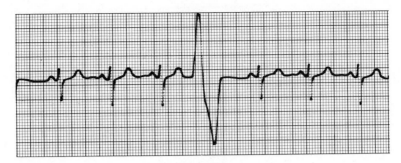

Fig. 8-3. Apparent full compensatory pause. Note that one P wave is obliterated by the anomalous complex, resulting in uncertainty as to whether there is a sinus P wave or a PAC.

proximate to the PVC because the ventricle is in a refractory period and thus unable to respond. There is, however, a response to the following P wave. This sequence causes what is called a full compensatory pause.

Notice that the P waves in Fig. 8-2 fall right on time in spite of the interruption of the normal ventricular rhythm by the PVC.

To measure a full compensatory pause, mark off three normal cycles. Then place the first mark on the P wave of the normal cycle preceding the PVC. The third mark should fall exactly on the P wave following the ventricular ectopic beat.

The full compensatory pause proves ventricular ectopy *only when the P wave proximal to it can be seen.* For example, in Fig. 8-2 the sinus P wave can be clearly seen in the T wave of the PVC. It is identified because it is on time with the sinus rhythm. In Fig. 8-3 there is a P wave lost within the PVC. Thus in this case you cannot be absolutely sure that it is there, even though the P wave following the PVC is on time. It could be that a PAC with aberrant ventricular conduction, discussed in Chapter 12, has occurred. If the PAC had suppressed the sinus node (overdrive suppression), then the P wave following the PVC would be delayed, simulating a full compensatory pause.

If an anomalous complex is *not* followed by a full compensatory pause, then one can be sure of atrial involvement; that is, a premature atrial complex has reset the sinus node (instead of suppressing it), causing the next sinus P wave to be early. This may also occur as a result of a PVC with retrograde conduction.

Increased amplitude

The greater amplitude usually demonstrated by the PVC is caused by a stronger vector, the result of a greater number of depolarized (negative) cells opposing polarized (positive) cells.

The normal cardiac vector passes along the anatomical axis of the heart, which is diagrammatically illustrated in Fig. 8-4.

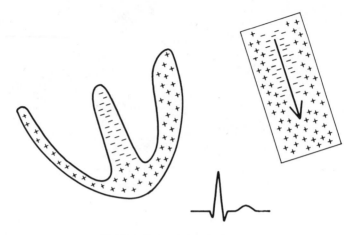

Fig. 8-4. Normal depolarization.

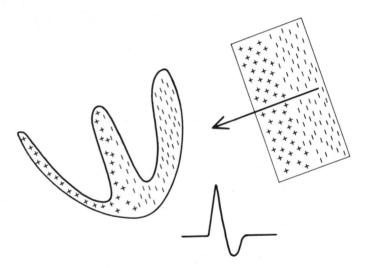

Fig. 8-5. Abnormal depolarization.

The usual sequence of electrical events in the heart causes an equalization of the electrical charges. The endocardium depolarizes before the epicardium. Thus there are fewer negative and positive charges opposing each other than would be the case if one half of the heart depolarized before the other half.

The vector from an ectopic focus often has a deviated axis (Fig. 8-5). One side of the heart, at the location of the ectopic focus, depolarizes before the other. This results in a greater number of negative cells in the presence of positive cells. The resultant stronger vector is reflected in the ECG tracing by a complex of higher amplitude than that of the dominant sinus rhythm.

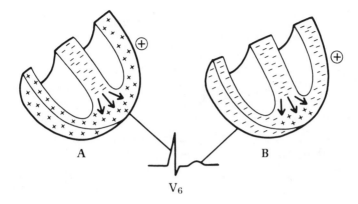

Fig. 8-6. A, Normal depolarization. **B,** Normal repolarization.

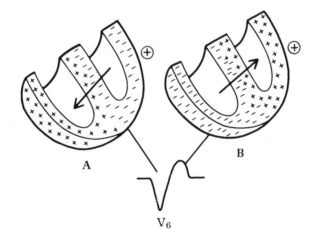

Fig. 8-7. A, Abnormal depolarization. **B,** Abnormal repolarization.

This strong vector of the PVC does not mean that the premature muscle contraction is stronger than normal. On the contrary, it is weaker because it occurs early, not allowing for complete ventricular filling, and because the contraction following this errant simulus is not uniform.

The compensatory pause following the PVC causes a longer ventricular filling time. Therefore the first normal beat following the PVC is more forceful.

T wave of opposite polarity

Normally repolarization occurs from epicardium to endocardium, beginning at the apex of the heart—just the opposite of the normal depolarization process (Fig. 8-6).

Since current flows from negative to positive, a normal repolarization process results in an upright T wave.

Conversely, the abnormal repolarization process follows the same sequence as did the abnormal depolarization process because, during delayed or abnormal depolarization, the cells at the apex are not activated soon enough to enable them to begin to repolarize first. Therefore the first cells to depolarize are the first cells to repolarize (Fig. 8-7).

Since the direction of the two processes (depolarization and repolarization) is the same, the polarity of the two deflections is opposite (the T wave is of opposite polarity to the terminal part of the QRS).

No related P wave

The ventricular ectopic impulse is not the result of atrial activity. Thus, although a P wave may immediately precede a PVC, it is not the cause of the ectopic ventricular activity.

TYPES OF PREMATURE VENTRICULAR CONTRACTIONS (PVCs)
End-diastolic PVC

If a ventricular ectopic beat occurs late in diastole, there is a P wave immediately preceding but unrelated to it. This P-R interval is shorter than the dominant P-R interval, and the ectopic complex may or may not be premature. This type of PVC is termed *end-diastolic* (Fig. 8-8) and is often a fusion beat (Chapter 14).

Because there is a normal P wave immediately preceding the end-diastolic PVC, it is frequently misdiagnosed as a PAC with aberrant ventricular conduction, but the ventricular complex, not the P wave, is premature.

Unifocal PVCs

Since the PVCs shown in Fig. 8-9 are identical in form, it is evident that they originate from a single focus in the ventricle.

PVC

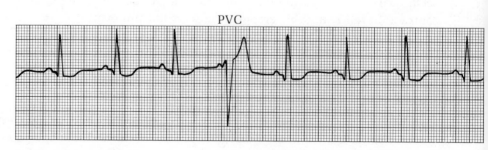

Fig. 8-8. End-diastolic premature ventricular contraction (PVC).

Ventricular bigeminy

Every other beat in the tracing shown in Fig. 8-10 is a PVC from the same focus. Each is coupled to the preceding normal complex.

Ventricular trigeminy

Ventricular trigeminy is a PVC characterized by rhythms that occur in groups of three. There may be one PVC for every two normal beats (Fig. 8-11) or two PVCs for each normal beat (Fig. 8-12).

Ventricular quadrigeminy

Fig. 8-13 is a tracing in which there are two ventricular ectopic beats for every two sinus-conducted complexes. When this pattern is repeated in any combination of four complexes, of which at least one is a ventricular ectopic beat, it is referred to as ventricular quadrigeminy.

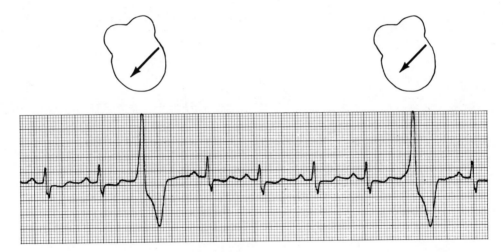

Fig. 8-9. Unifocal PVCs.

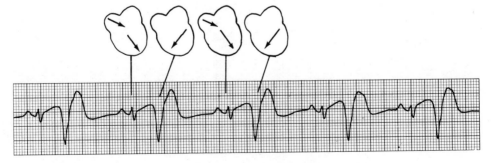

Fig. 8-10. Ventricular bigeminy.

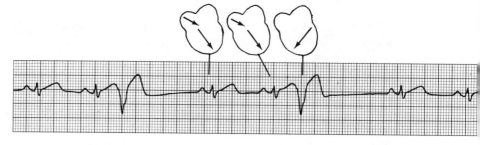

Fig. 8-11. Ventricular trigeminy, two normal complexes and one PVC.

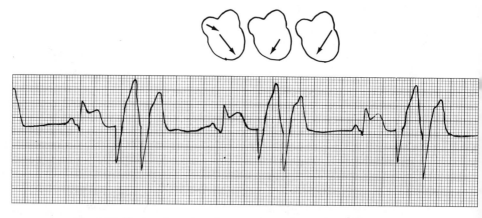

Fig. 8-12. Ventricular trigeminy, one normal complex and two PVCs.

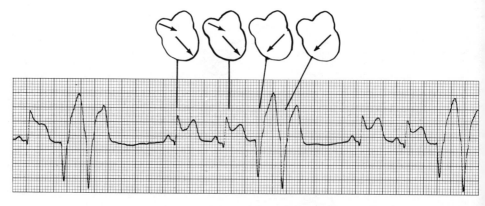

Fig. 8-13. Ventricular quadrigeminy.

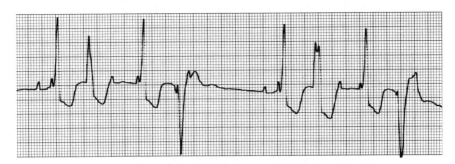

Fig. 8-14. Multifocal PVCs.

PVCs WITH MORE SERIOUS IMPLICATIONS

Ventricular ectopic beats occurring in a diseased heart constitute a serious condition. There are, however, degrees of seriousness. Frequent, multifocal, left ventricular, and/or paired PVCs are more ominous than the occasional unifocal ventricular extrasystole. A PVC occurring during the relative refractory or vulnerable period would be even more ominous.

Multifocal PVCs

In the tracing shown in Fig. 8-14 there are two, and perhaps 3, distinct contours to the PVCs (second, fourth, sixth, and eighth complexes) indicating that in each case the vector is oriented differently to the axis of the lead. The ventricles have more than one ectopic focus. The second and sixth complexes are also interpolated and are followed by concealed retrograde conduction as evidenced by the long P-Rs.

Paired PVCs

The PVCs in Fig. 8-15 occur in pairs, or *back to back.* There is a very real danger that the second of the pair will meet with refractory tissue and result in electrical chaos, or ventricular fibrillation.

R-on-T phenomenon

The term *R-on-T phenomenon* is used to indicate that an R wave (PVC) has occurred during the relative refractory period (on the T wave). Because the heart is not yet ready to respond to this stimulus in an organized fashion, a serious ventricular arrhythmia may result.

In Fig. 8-16 a PVC has occurred during the vulnerable period (on the T wave).

Again, in the same patient, Fig. 8-17 illustrates a PVC that falls on the T wave. The premature vector has stimulated a partially repolarized ventricle and has met with both nonrefractory and refractory tissue, resulting in ventricular fibrillation.

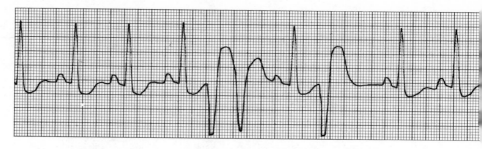

Fig. 8-15. Paired PVCs.

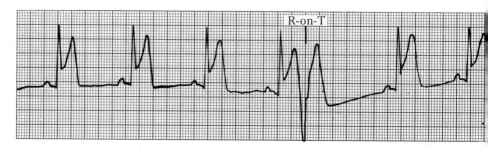

Fig. 8-16. R-on-T phenomenon.

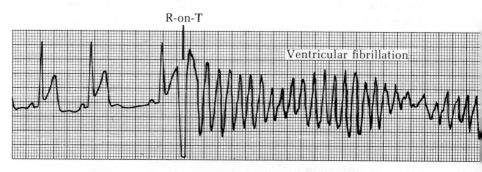

Fig. 8-17. R-on-T phenomenon causing ventricular fibrillation.

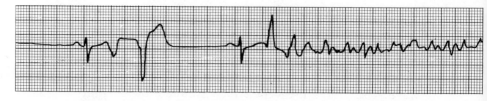

Fig. 8-18. Paired multifocal PVCs resulting in ventricular fibrillation.

Fig. 8-18 shows a marked sinus bradycardia with coupled multifocal PVCs occurring on the T wave and resulting finally in ventricular fibrillation.

Left ventricular PVC

Ventricular ectopic beats that arise in the left ventricle are more serious than those arising in the right ventricle. The origin of the ectopic beat can be determined by the direction of the complex in V_1.

An ectopic vector proceeding from a focus in the left ventricle would travel toward the positive electrode of V_1, causing a positive deflection (Fig. 8-19).

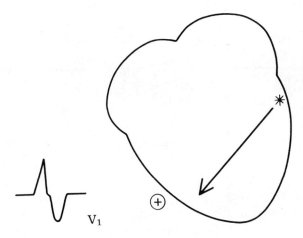

Fig. 8-19. Left ventricular PVC.

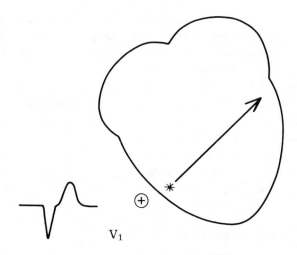

Fig. 8-20. Right ventricular PVC.

V_1

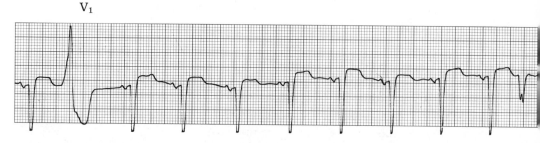

Fig. 8-21. In V_1 a left ventricular PVC is positive (second complex) and a right ventricular PVC is negative (last complex).

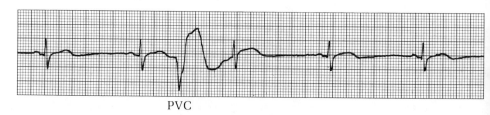

PVC

Fig. 8-22. Interpolated PVC.

An ectopic vector proceeding from a focus in the right ventricle would travel away from the positive electrode of V_1, causing a negative deflection (Fig. 8-20). Fig. 8-21 illustrates left and right ventricular PVCs in one tracing.

EXCEPTIONS TO THE RULES

Ventricular extrasystoles are generally most easily recognized because of their full compensatory pause and the broadened complex that is much different in appearance from the normal sinus-conducted complexes. There are, however, exceptions to these rules. Two types of ventricular extrasystoles are not followed by the full compensatory pause. They are the interpolated extrasystole and the extrasystole with retrograde conduction to the atria. But in the latter case, if the ectopic depolarization of the atria has suppressed the sinus node, then a full compensatory pause is simulated. There is also a type that has a normal or almost normal appearance. If the ectopic focus is in one of the fascicles (fascicular ectopic), then the resultant complex may be only a little broader and may differ mainly because of an axis shift.

Interpolated extrasystole

This PVC is interposed (interpolated between two normal sinus beats) without disturbing the basic rhythm. The sinus node discharges normally,

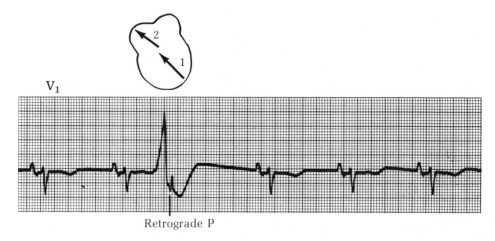

Retrograde P

Fig. 8-23. PVC with retrograde conduction to the atria.

and the expected ventricular response is undisturbed. The interpolated extrasystole occurs only when the basic rate is so slow that it is physiologically possible to find the myocardium nonrefractory long enough to complete the response to an ectopic stimulus and return to the nonrefractory state before the next expected normal ventricular response.

The basic rate in the tracing shown in Fig. 8-22 is 47. In response to an ectopic stimulus the ventricles are able to depolarize, repolarize, and return to a nonrefractory state before the next expected normal beat. Since the ventricular rhythm is uninterrupted, the interpolated PVC does not have a full compensatory pause.

Ventricular extrasystole with retrograde conduction

In most cases the depolarization current from the ectopic focus in the ventricle does not travel up the AV junction to activate the atrium (retrograde conduction). When it does, the sinus node is depolarized early, and the next normal sinus stimulus occurs a little earlier than normal. This sequence of events produces a less than full compensatory pause.

Fig. 8-23 is a tracing in which a P′ wave can be seen immediately following the PVC. In leads II, III, and aV_F, retrograde activation of the atria causes a negative P′ wave. The lead illustrated here is V_1, in which case the retrograde P′ wave is not necessarily negative.

Fascicular ectopics

Ectopic beats originating in the posterior fascicle of the left bundle branch would have left axis deviation, and those originating in the anterior fascicle would have right axis deviation. Figs. 8-24 and 8-25 illustrate the mechanism and the ECG as seen in the bipolar limb leads.

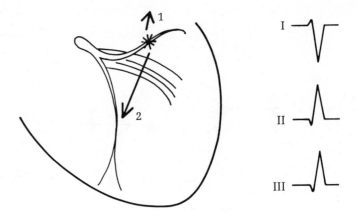

Fig. 8-24. Complexes produced in the bipolar limb leads from an ectopic focus in the anterior fascicle of the LBB.

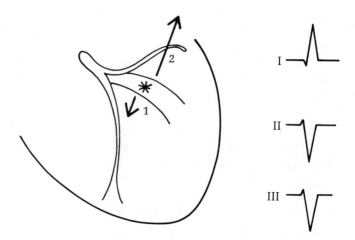

Fig. 8-25. Complexes produced in the bipolar limb leads from an ectopic focus in the posterior fascicle of the LBB.

Ventricular tachycardia

In ventricular tachycardia due either to a reentry mechanism within the His-Purkinje system or to an area of increased automaticity, the ECG shows a continuous series of broad, rapid ventricular ectopic beats (Fig. 8-26). In acute MI sustained ventricular tachycardia is rare. It either deteriorates into ventricular fibrillation or terminates.

PAROXYSMAL VENTRICULAR TACHYCARDIA

Paroxysmal ventricular tachycardia is a burst of tachycardia initiated by a PVC. In Fig. 8-27, eleven PVCs follow the initial premature beat, after

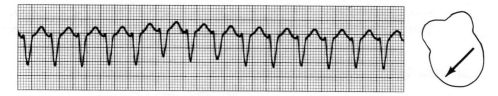

Fig. 8-26. Ventricular tachycardia.

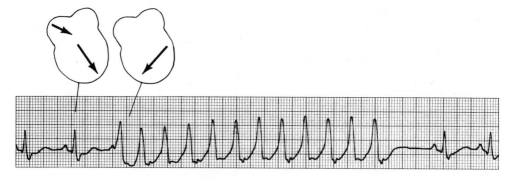

Fig. 8-27. Paroxysmal ventricular tachycardia with 2:1 retrograde conduction.

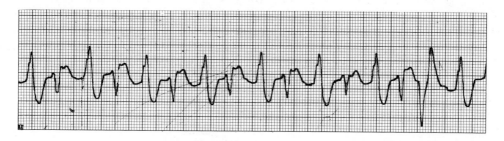

Fig. 8-28. Bidirectional ventricular tachycardia.

which the tachycardia is terminated and the sinus node is once again in command. Paroxysmal ventricular tachycardia, then, is a series of PVCs that ends spontaneously. Note in this tracing the 2:1 retrograde conduction to the atria. In every other T wave a retrograde P' can be seen.

BIDIRECTIONAL VENTRICULAR TACHYCARDIA

Fig. 8-28 illustrates bidirectional ventricular tachycardia. His bundle recordings have confirmed that both types of beats in this arrhythmia originate in the ventricles. On the frontal plane leads there is alternating left and right axis deviation with an underlying right bundle branch block. When digitalis intoxication goes unrecognized past the stage of the accelerated junctional rhythm, this arrhythmia is frequently next and may be a terminal event.

Ventricular fibrillation

Ventricular fibrillation involves electrical activity that is not unified. Individual muscle fibers are depolarizing, but they are disorganized and fail to produce a proper ventricular contraction. The heart quivers and twitches (Fig. 8-29).

The electrodes record this erratic activity, as shown in Fig. 8-30. Coarse ventricular fibrillation (Fig. 8-30, *A*) indicates more electrical activity in the ventricles and is easier to convert than a fine ventricular fibrillation (Fig. 8-30, *B*).

In Fig. 8-31 a very rapid ventricular tachycardia (ventricular flutter) where the QRS and T are merged indistinguishably deteriorates into ventricular fibrillation.

Accelerated idioventricular rhythm

When an area of enhanced automaticity within the ventricles paces the heart at a rate less than 100 beats/min and yet more than the inherent rate of ventricular pacemaker cells, the rhythm is sometimes called an accelerated idioventricular rhythm. This arrhythmia is often seen accompanying acute myocardial infarction and was initially thought to be benign. However, clinical experience has shown that life-threatening arrhythmias can be precipitated by the accelerated idioventricular focus.

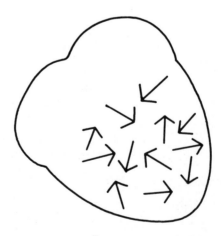

Fig. 8-29. Disorganized electrical activity of ventricular fibrillation.

An area of enhanced automaticity within the ventricular conductive system need only be greater than 40 beats/min to be considered accelerated. Thus this arrhythmia often does not manifest itself at all until its rate exceeds that of the sinus node. Then, because its rate is so similar to that of the sinus node, it usually begins and ends with fusion beats (pp. 168 to 171). This is the case in Fig. 8-32 where the sinus rate is 53 and the rate of the ventricular focus is 52. When the rate of the sinus node slows down slightly, there is a fusion beat; that is, the sinus impulse enters the ventricles at about the same time that the ventricular ectopic focus discharges. The result is a collision of forces within the ventricles, producing a complex that is not ex-

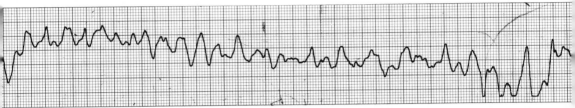

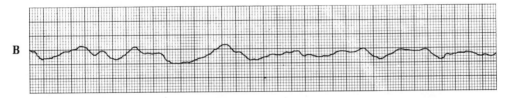

Fig. 8-30. Ventricular fibrillation. **A,** With a coarse fibrillatory line. **B,** With a fine fibrillatory line.

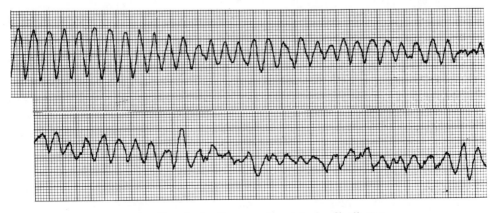

Fig. 8-31. Ventricular flutter and ventricular fibrillation.

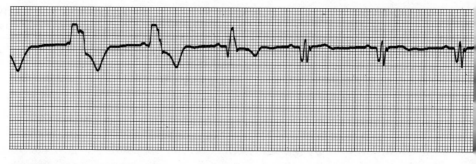

Fig. 8-32. Accelerated idioventricular rhythm with a rate of 52. The sinus rate is 53. Note tha the third complex is a fusion beat.

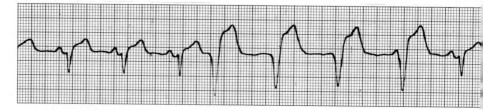

Fig. 8-33. Accelerated idioventricular rhythm with a rate of 67 and an underlying normal sinus rhythm.

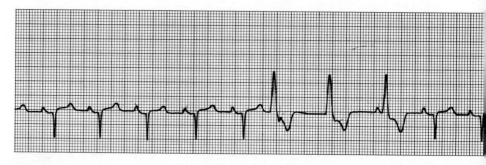

Fig. 8-34. Accelerated idioventricular rhythm with a rate of 74 beats/min. The sinus rate is 86 beats/min.

actly like the sinus-conducted beats or exactly like the pure ectopic beat. The third complex in Fig. 8-32 is a fusion beat.

Fig. 8-33 illustrates another accelerated idioventricular rhythm. This time the ventricular ectopic focus takes over in the face of an adequate sinus rhythm and normal AV conduction. Although the rate of the ectopic focus is only 67, it is still too fast for a ventricular pacemaker. Some authorities believe that this type of an accelerated idioventricular rhythm should be treated more aggressively because the ectopic rhythm asserted itself when there was no default in sinus performance or AV conduction and because the first of the ectopic beats is so premature.

Fig. 8-34 illustrates another accelerated idioventricular rhythm that takes over very prematurely, in the face of an adequate sinus rate of 86 beats/min. This tracing has no fusion beats.

Ventricular parasystole

In this arrhythmia there is an area of enhanced automaticity within the ventricular conductive system that is protected from the basic rhythm by *entrance block*. Thus it maintains its own uninterrupted rate of discharge, being undisturbed by the basic rhythm. Sometimes the impulse does not emerge from its focus even when the ventricles are nonrefractory. This is called *exit block*. Entrance and exit block will now be described.

ENTRANCE AND EXIT BLOCKS

One of the effects of ischemia on the myocardial cells is the reduction of the resting membrane potential and the resultant decremental conduction.

Reduction of the resting membrane potential lowers the rate of rise and the amplitude of the action potential. The amplitude of the action potential determines the conduction velocity. Therefore it is possible that a group of cells in the His-Purkinje system which have lost their normal resting membrane potential are able to spread weak but effective depolarization currents to adjacent cells (decremental conduction) but are unable to be depolarized from an external stimulus (entrance block). It may also happen that the current is too weak to be conducted to neighboring cells (exit block).

ECG changes

1. The ectopic complexes are not accurately coupled to the sinus beats; that is, they are independent of the sinus mechanism and do not require preceding activity for their initiation.
2. Fusion beats sometimes occur, indicating independent ectopic activity.
3. Since the rhythm of the ectopic focus is regular, the time interval between the parasystolic complexes is often but not necessarily always constant. The ectopic focus depolarizes regularly but may not manifest a complex each time due to refractory ventricular tissue. Therefore the longest ectopic interval may be divisible by the shortest ectopic interval, indicating a regular rhythm.

When interectopic intervals with exact multiples are not found, this does not exclude the parasystolic focus, since the conduction times from the ectopic focus to the ventricular myocardium may vary. Such would be the case if Wenckebach conduction were present in the tissue surrounding the ectopic

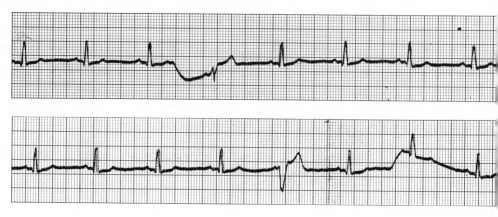

Fig. 8-35. Ventricular parasystole

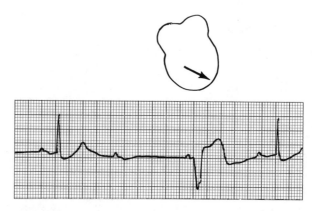

Fig. 8-36. Ventricular escape due to AV conduction block.

focus. The coupling intervals of the PVCs in Fig. 8-35 are different in each case. The shortest interval between ectopic beats (the last two) may be evenly divided into the longest interval, indicating that the ectopic focus is undisturbed by the sinus-conducted ventricular impulses. The absence of fixed coupling indicates that the ventricular ectopic beat is not due to reentry; that is, first and last ectopic beats are fusion beats, further confirming the independence of the ectopic focus.

Ventricular escape

When rhythmic impulses from the sinus node are no longer being transmitted into the ventricles, a lower pacemaker, usually in the bundle of His, manifests its own inherent rhythm at a rate of 40 to 60 beats/min. The ventricles are then paced at this rate independently of the atria. This is a passive

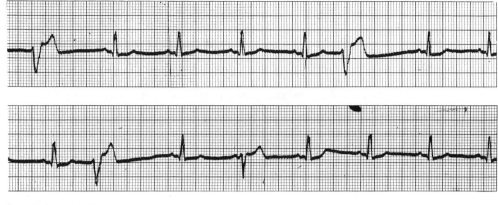

(continuous strips).

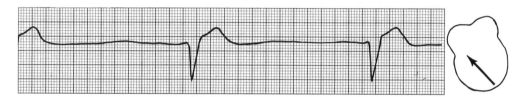

Fig. 8-37. Slow idioventricular rhythm.

mechanism known as ventricular escape. Fig. 8-36 depicts the failure of the sinus node to conduct impulses to the ventricle. After two nonconducted P waves there is ventricular escape. The escape beat is broad, indicating that the focus is below the bifurcation of the bundle of His.

SLOW IDIOVENTRICULAR RHYTHM

In Fig. 8-37 the ventricular rate is 23, and the QRS complexes are broad (0.20 sec). This is evidence of a pacemaker low in the conductive system. No P waves are apparent. They may be seen in another lead, or they may be truly absent, in which case there is atrial standstill with an idioventricular rhythm.

Summary

Ectopic foci in the ventricles usually originate in the conductive system as a result of reentry and/or enhanced automaticity, but they may possibly also originate outside the conductive system as a result of afterpotentials. PVCs may result in the more serious arrhythmias of ventricular tachycardia or ventricular fibrillation.

An accelerated idioventricular rhythm has a rate that is less than 100 beats/min but greater than the inherent rate of the ventricular conductive system. It commonly begins and ends with fusion beats.

A parasystolic focus is an area of enhanced automaticity, protected from the basic rhythm by entrance block.

Ventricular escape beats and rhythms are the normal response of the ventricular conductive system to a lack of stimulus from faster pacemakers.

CHAPTER 9

Heart block

Heart block is classified as either first, second, or third degree. In first-degree heart block all sinus impulses are conducted, but the conduction time is prolonged. In second-degree heart block some of the sinus impulses are not conducted, and in third-degree heart block none of the sinus impulses are conducted.

Incidence of heart block in myocardial infarction

From 7% to 10% of all patients with acute myocardial infarction have first-degree heart block, 5% have second-degree heart block, and 5% to 6% have complete (third-degree) heart block. The block is usually a transient condition, and normal sinus rhythm will be restored within 2 weeks in 90% of patients.

First-degree AV block

First-degree AV block may be caused by a conduction delay anywhere from the atria to the ventricles. It manifests itself in a long P-R interval. The impulse from the sinus node is propagated in all beats but is delayed either as it traverses the AV junction or within the atria, resulting in a P-R interval of over 0.20 sec.

In the tracing shown in Fig. 9-1 all P waves are conducted, but the P-R interval is too long (0.36 sec). The QRS interval is slightly prolonged.

In Fig. 9-2 the P-R interval is too long (0.24 sec), and the QRS interval is normal (0.10 sec).

Second-degree AV block

Second-degree heart block is characterized by nonconducted P waves and is generally classified into type I (Wenckebach) and type II.

SECOND-DEGREE HEART BLOCK, TYPE I (Wenckebach)

Type I second-degree heart block is characterized by the cyclic noncon-duction of P waves that terminates a period of increasingly prolonged P-R

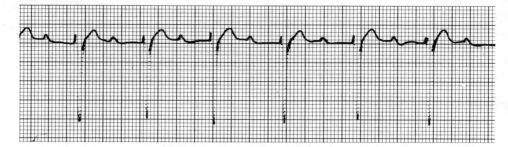

Fig. 9-1. First-degree heart block.

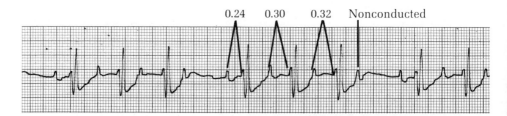

Fig. 9-2. First-degree heart block.

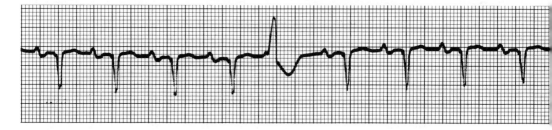

0.28   0.38   0.40   Nonconducted

Fig. 9-3. Second-degree heart block, type I (Wenckebach) with a narrow QRS.

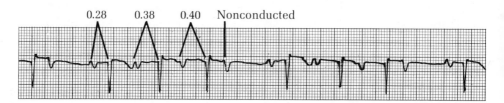

0.24   0.30   0.32   Nonconducted

Fig. 9-4. Second-degree heart block, type I (Wenckebach) with a broad QRS.

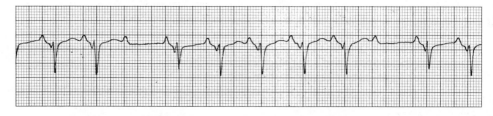

Fig. 9-5. Second-degree heart block, type II.

intervals. The QRS complexes are usually narrow, since the conduction delay commonly occurs within the AV node.

The classic Wenckebach pattern has lengthening P-R intervals, shortening R-R intervals, and a pause that is less than twice the shortest cycle. The ventricular complexes occur at shorter intervals because the greatest increment in the P-R intervals is between the first and second P-R intervals. Notice that in Fig. 9-3 the first P-R is 0.28 sec and the second increases by 0.10 sec whereas the increase in the third P-R interval is only another 0.02 sec. This causes a shortening of the R-R intervals. Atypical Wenckebach patterns are also commonly seen, in which case these rules do not apply. If the greatest increment occurs in the third or fourth P-R interval instead of in the second, then the first R-R interval is not the longest of the group.

Fig. 9-3 shows the cyclic and gradual increase of the P-R interval until the last P wave of the group is not conducted. The first P-R interval beginning the cycle is 0.28 sec. The second is 0.38 sec and PR 3, 0.40 sec. The fourth P wave is not conducted. When three sinus complexes are conducted and one is not, the conduction ratio is said to be 4:3.

The gradual and progressive slowing of the impulse propagation seen in the Wenckebach phenomenon usually occurs within the AV node. As the con-

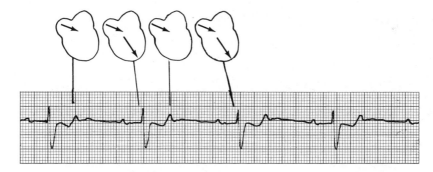

Fig. 9-6. Second-degree heart block with 2:1 AV conduction and a broad QRS.

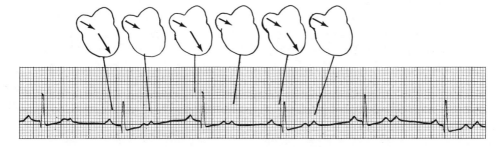

Fig. 9-7. Second-degree heart block with 2:1 AV conduction and a narrow QRS.

duction velocity decreases, the refractory period lengthens, causing the P waves to fall closer and closer to this refractory period until it becomes inevitable that a P wave will eventually be nonconducted.

Of less common occurrence is the Wenckebach phenomenon associated with broad QRS complexes, as seen in Fig. 9-4. The AV conduction disturbance is thought to be at two levels. In the AV node it accounts for the increments in P-R intervals. In both bundle branches, conduction disturbance is reflected in the wide QRS. However, it has been shown that the Wenckebach phenomenon may also be a manifestation of block in the bundle of His or where it branches (H-V).

SECOND-DEGREE HEART BLOCK, TYPE II

In type II second-degree heart block the nonconducted P wave is seen against a background of P-R intervals that are all the same (Fig. 9-5). These intervals may or may not be prolonged. It is important to compare the P-R intervals before and after the nonconducted beat. If there is a measurable difference, then the tracing is difficult to classify, and further investigations are indicated to define exactly whether it is type I or type II.

Treatment and prognosis are governed by the level of the conduction delay within the AV junction. A broadened QRS complex indicates a more ominous anatomical lesion.

DIFFERENTIAL DIAGNOSIS BETWEEN TYPE I AND TYPE II AV BLOCK

In second-degree heart block, when there are not two conducted beats in a row, it is impossible to distinguish with certainty between type I and type II AV block on the ECG. Figs. 9-6 and 9-7 are examples of this. In both tracings the conduction ratio is 2:1 (two P waves for every QRS); therefore it is impossible to know whether or not the P-R interval would have lengthened if two consecutive P waves had been conducted.

In Fig. 9-6 the marked lengthening of the P-R interval is thought to indicate AV nodal disease, since conduction decrements in the AV node are more easily detected on the ECG than they are in the conductive system below the AV node.

When the P-R intervals before the dropped beat are all the same, close attention should be paid to the P-R interval after the dropped beat. Sufficiently long rhythm strips may reveal a shortening of the P-R interval after the nonconducted P wave and thus an atypical type I second-degree block.

It should also be noted that nonconducted P waves may also be produced by a concealed junctional premature beat. In such a situation the junctional ectopic would discharge and depolarize the AV junction but be blocked in both antegrade and retrograde directions. This beat would not be seen on the

ECG and is therefore called *concealed*. The AV junction would be refractory, and the next P wave would be nonconducted.

Complete (third-degree) heart block

The sole muscular channel for the propagation of the electrical impulse from atria to ventricles is the AV junction. If there is a lesion serious enough to block conduction at any level in the junction, complete AV heart block results.

Complete heart block can result from lesions in one or more of the three sites illustrated in Fig. 9-8: the AV node, bundle of His, and right and left bundle branches (trifascicular block).

In complete heart block the rate and dependability of the ventricular rhythm is related to the level of the lesion. A pacemaker at the top of the bundle of His has a rate of about 50 and is relatively dependable. However, if the pacemaker is at the branching segment of the bundle of His, the rate is slower and less dependable.

The P waves in Fig. 9-9 can be seen to occur regularly at a rate of 100. They are totally independent of the ventricular rate of 46. The sinus node paces the atria, and the AV junction paces the ventricles. Since the QRS complex is of normal duration (0.08 sec), the ventricular pacemaker must be above the bifurcation of the bundle of His. This is called an *idiojunctional rhythm*.

The diagnosis of this arrhythmia is straightforward. Walking out the P waves and R waves shows two independent pacemakers. In spite of this, an

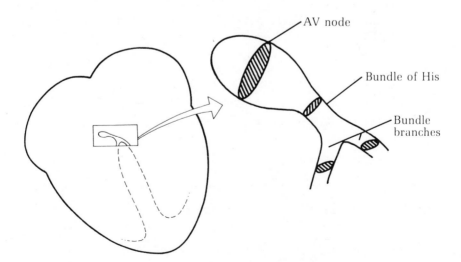

Fig. 9-8. The three possible sites of lesions in complete heart block.

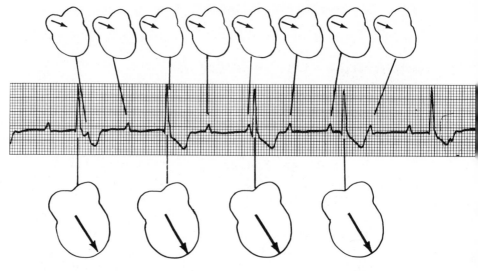

Fig. 9-9. Complete heart block with an idiojunctional rhythm.

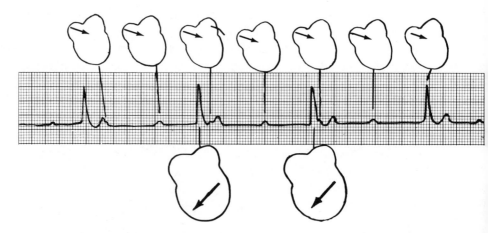

Fig. 9-10. Complete heart block with an idioventricular rhythm.

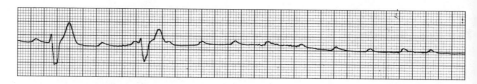

Fig. 9-11. Complete heart block with a failing ventricular pacemaker.

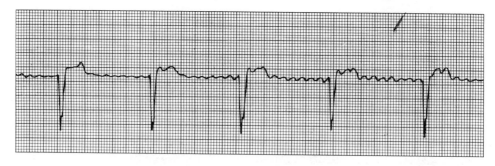

Fig. 9-12. Atrial fibrillation with complete heart block.

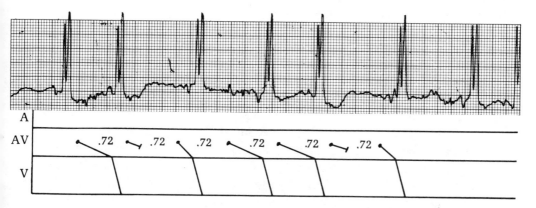

Fig. 9-13. Atrial fibrillation with complete heart block, junctional tachycardia, and Wenckebach conduction.

error is commonly made. After glancing briefly at the tracing, you might say that it is second-degree heart block with 2:1 AV block, but if that were the situation, the P-R intervals of the conducted beats would all be the same.

The P waves occur at a rate of 75 in Fig. 9-10. They are regular and undisturbed by the ventricular rhythm of 36. This is complete heart block with an *idioventricular rhythm.* The broad QRS complex (0.12 sec) indicates a focus below the branching of the bundle of His.

Fig. 9-11 shows complete heart block when the ventricular pacemaker fails, resulting in ventricular asystole.

Complete heart block in atrial fibrillation

The ventricular response to atrial fibrillation should normally be irregular. When it is not, pathological heart block or digitalis toxicity should be suspected. In Fig. 9-12 complete heart block is reflected by a regular idiojunctional rhythm in the presence of atrial fibrillation. Digitalis acts to increase the refractory period in the AV node. Toxic blood levels cause AV block.

The heart block is not so apparent in Fig. 9-13. At first glance it appears to be atrial fibrillation with an appropriately irregular ventricular response. However, there is group beating, the first clue to the Wenckebach phenomenon. Groups of three with shortening R-R intervals and a pause that is twice the shortest cycle are all signs of Wenckebach. Laddergrams are not discussed until the next chapter; however, one is helpful here to illustrate the mechanism of this arrhythmia: complete heart block and atrial fibrillation, along with junctional tachycardia. Although the junctional pacemaker is firing at a rate of 79, there is Wenckebach conduction in which every third beat is not conducted (Wenckebach 3 : 2). The heart block, junctional tachycardia, and Wenckebach conduction are all manifestations of digitalis toxicity, and may be seen as well in the postoperative cardiac patient and those with myocarditis.

Summary

In first-degree AV block the P-R interval is prolonged beyond 0.20 sec. In second-degree AV block the P-R interval may be either normal or prolonged, but some impulses are not conducted to the ventricles. In complete heart block (third-degree AV block) the atria and ventricles beat separately. The atria are usually paced by the sinus node at a normal rate, and the ventricles are paced by the His-Purkinje system. A pacemaker above the bifurcation of the bundle of His produces what is called an idiojunctional rhythm. A pacemaker below the bundle of His produces an idioventricular rhythm. The rate of an idioventricular pacemaker in complete heart block is usually not above 40 beats/min.

CHAPTER 10

Laddergrams: how and when to use them

Laddergrams are graphic displays of the chronological conduction events within the heart. Fig. 10-1 illustrates how the sections of the heart are displayed on the graph. The first small section is reserved for the activity of the sinus node and is used only when there is a conduction problem between the sinus node and the atrial muscle, such as would occur with Wenckebach of the sinus node. The second section represents the atria; the last section represents the ventricles, with the AV junctional area between the two.

Laddergrams are useful in explaining some of the more complex arrhythmias when it may otherwise be difficult to illustrate the underlying mechanism. They are hardly of use when the mechanism is obvious and straightforward. Apart from their value as a teaching tool, they are surprisingly helpful when one is presented with a rhythm strip, the mechanism of which is not readily apparent. In these situations, to simply begin the laddergram, marking out what is known about the arrhythmia, is the first step toward understanding the mechanism.

How to begin

Begin the laddergram by marking off what is seen on the tracing. A ruler lines up the beginning of the P waves with the appropriate tier in the laddergram. This atrial line may be straight down from the beginning of the P wave, as is illustrated in this book, or it may slant toward the end of the P wave. The ventricular complexes are then drawn in the third tier. In supraventricular rhythms this line should be slanted with the leading point at the top of the tier and coinciding with the beginning of the ventricular complex. The end of the ventricular complex is marked at the bottom of the tier, and the slanted line drawn between the two marks (*V* in Fig. 10-2, *A*). The next step, illustrated in Fig. 10-2, *B*, consists of indicating AV conduction by connecting the bottom of the atrial line with the top of the ventricular line.

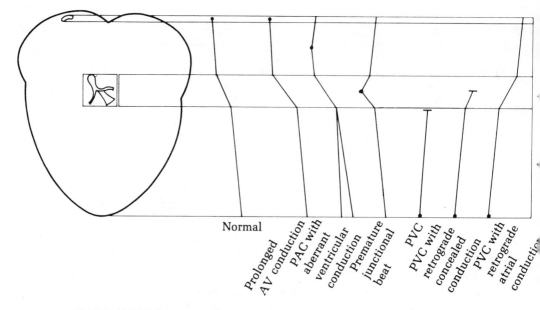

Fig. 10-1. (From Conover, M. H.: Cardiac arrhythmias: exercises in pattern interpretation, ed. 2, St. Louis, 1978, The C. V. Mosby Co.)

Ventricular ectopics

If the ventricular complex is ectopic, the leading point of the laddergram should be at the bottom of the ventricular tier at a point coinciding with the beginning of the ventricular ectopic complex. A line would then be drawn forward and up to a point at the top of the tier coinciding with the end of the ventricular ectopic complex. A normal sinus-conducted complex and a PVC are shown in Fig. 10-3.

PACs

Fig. 10-4 illustrates a normal sinus-conducted beat and a PAC with normal ventricular conduction. Notice that the leading point of the laddergram is not at the top of the atrial tier but in the middle, indicating that the pacemaker of this particular complex was not the sinus node but an ectopic focus.

Retrograde conduction

A PVC with retrograde conduction to the atria is shown in Fig. 10-5, with the leading point at the bottom of the graph to indicate a ventricular ectopic focus. The chronological order of conduction is then illustrated by the slant

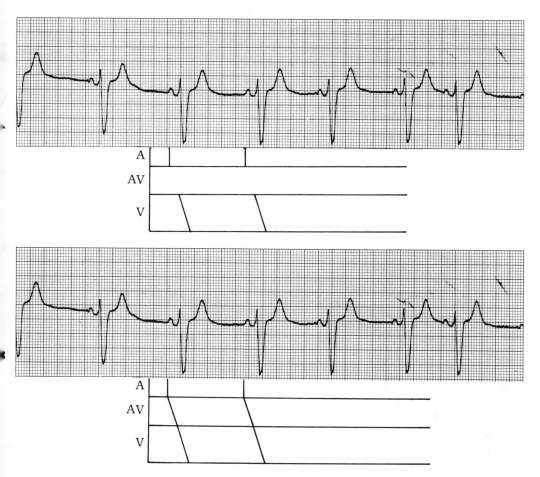

Fig. 10-2. A, First step: draw lines indicating intra-atrial and intraventricular conduction. **B,** Second step: draw lines indicating AV conduction.

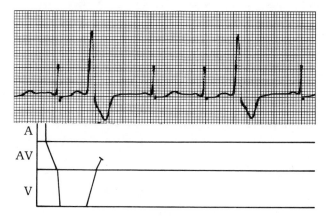

Fig. 10-3. Normal sinus-conducted beat and a PVC.

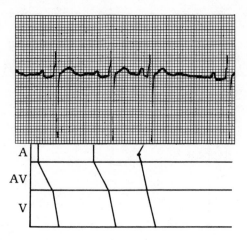

Fig. 10-4. Two normal sinus-conducted beats and a PAC.

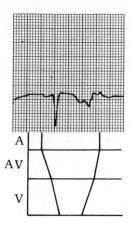

Fig. 10-5. Normal sinus-conducted beat and a PVC with retrograde conduction to the atria.

of the line from the bottom to the top through the AV junctional tier and retrogradely into the atria.

Junctional rhythms

The junctional tachycardia in Fig. 10-6 is interrupted by one sinus P wave that conducts to the ventricles. The junctional rhythm has retrograde conduction to the atria. This is illustrated with the leading point of the ladder-gram placed in the AV junctional tier at a point before the beginning of the P′ wave. A line is drawn forward and up toward the P′ wave and then retro-gradely into the atrial tier. Sometimes arrows are used to more clearly illus-

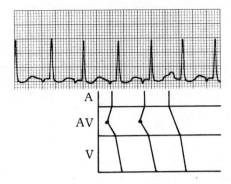

Fig. 10-6. Junctional tachycardia and a normal sinus-conducted beat.

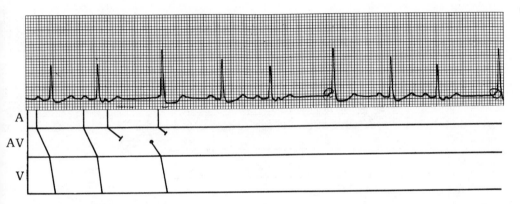

Fig. 10-7. Two normal sinus-conducted beats, followed by a nonconducted PAC, a junctional escape beat, and a nonconducted sinus P wave.

trate the direction of conduction. A line is then drawn forward and down to the point in the ventricular tier coinciding with the beginning of the ventricular complex. Anterograde conduction through the ventricles is then indicated by a line that proceeds to the bottom of the tier to a point that corresponds to the end of the ventricular complex.

Conduction blocks and escape beats

Fig. 10-7 illustrates a nonconducted PAC, followed by a junctional escape beat that coincides with a sinus P wave. The junctional escape beat is drawn by starting the graph in the AV junctional tier at an appropriate point before the beginning of the junctional complex. The actual depolarization of the junctional pacemaker site is not seen on the surface ECG. A slanted line is

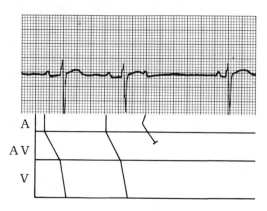

Fig. 10-8. Two normal sinus-conducted beats and a nonconducted PAC.

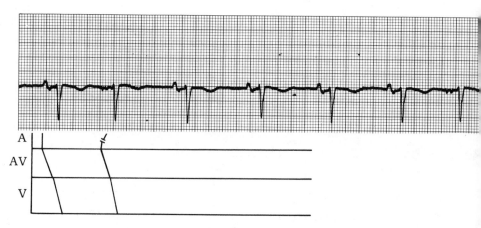

Fig. 10-9. Normal sinus-conducted beat and atrial fusion.

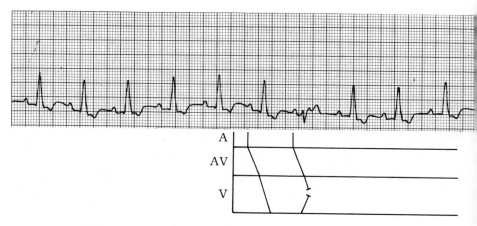

Fig. 10-10. Normal sinus-conducted beat and ventricular fusion.

then drawn from the selected point to the top of the ventricular tier at the place just below where the junctional complex begins. The sinus P wave can be seen distorting the onset of the junctional complex.

Fig. 10-8 is another illustration of a nonconducted PAC. The ectopic P wave is indicated as previously described, and then a line is slanted into the AV tier and shown to end in a block.

Fusion

Figs. 10-9 and 10-10 illustrate atrial and ventricular fusion beats. The collision of electrical forces producing the fusion beat can be nicely depicted in the laddergram.

Wenckebach phenomenon

The lengthening AV conduction and the nonconducted beat of the Wenckebach phenomenon are illustrated in Fig. 10-11. Notice that although at a glance the ECG appears to have an irregular sinus rhythm, the laddergram clearly shows that the sinus rhythm is regular and the AV conduction time is lengthening. The arrhythmia shown is Wenckebach 3:2.

Reciprocal beats and rhythms

Probably one of the most useful purposes for the laddergram is to illustrate the reciprocating rhythm. Fig. 10-12 illustrates a PAC that is followed by normal ventricular conduction. This early impulse causes disunity in the AV node and, although it enters the ventricles normally, it goes back up the nonrefractory side of the AV node to produce an atrial echo beat. This im-

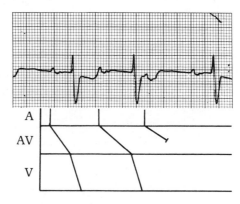

Fig. 10-11. Wenckebach conduction.

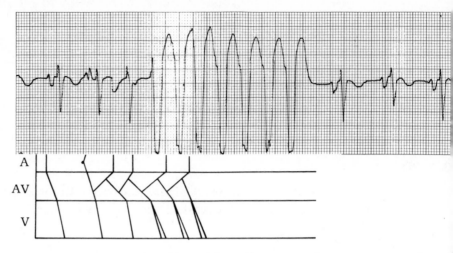

Fig. 10-12. Normal sinus-conducted beat, followed by a PAC and a reciprocating tachycard[...] with aberrant ventricular conduction.

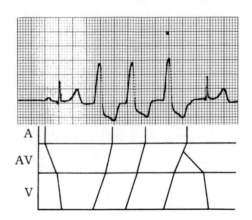

Fig. 10-13. Normal sinus-conducted beat, followed by PVCs with retrograde Wenckebach co[...] duction and a reciprocal beat. (From Conover, M. H.: Cardiac arrhythmias: exercises in patte[...] interpretation, ed. 2, St. Louis, 1978, The C. V. Mosby Co.)

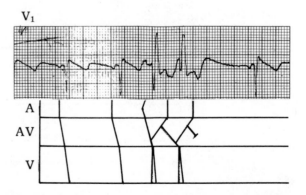

Fig. 10-14. Two normal sinus-conducted beats followed by a PAC and two reciprocal beats w[...] aberrant ventricular conduction.

pulse is again transmitted down the other side of the AV node, which is now nonrefractory and produces an almost normal ventricular complex, known as a reciprocal beat. The sequence continues in a reciprocating rhythm, with all but two of the ventricular complexes reflecting LBBB aberration.

A reciprocal beat is again illustrated in Fig. 10-13. This time it follows three PVCs that have retrograde Wenckebach conduction to the atria. Note the lengthening R-P intervals. The third P' wave of the series is followed by antegrade conduction to the ventricles and normal conduction (a reciprocal beat).

The laddergram in Fig. 10-14 illustrates the reciprocating mechanism initiated by a PAC. RBBB aberration is apparent in this burst of supraventricular tachycardia.

Aberrant ventricular conduction is covered in Chapter 12. Reciprocating (AV nodal reentry) mechanisms are covered in Chapter 3.

CHAPTER 11

Bundle branch block and hemiblock

One of the most distinctive examples of an intraventricular conduction defect is the obstruction of impulse conduction in one of the bundle branches

Ordinarily, the two lateral walls of the ventricles depolarize at almost the same time (Fig. 11-1). The current reaches both bundles at the same time and the entire ventricular muscle is depolarized.

An obstruction in either of the bundle branches would cause the affected side to be depolarized late (Figs. 11-2 and 11-3). This delay in the process of depolarization results in a distorted QRS complex of 0.12 sec or more in duration. Additionally, the T wave is opposite in polarity to the terminal part of the QRS.

Normal ventricular activation time (VAT)

The length of time required for the depolarization wave to travel from the endocardium to the epicardium is called the *ventricular activation time,* or

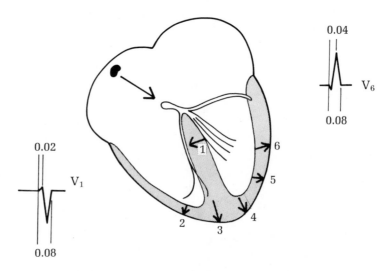

Fig. 11-1. Normal ventricular depolarization as reflected in V_1 and V_6.

VAT. It normally reaches its peak in the left ventricle because the left ventricle is larger and takes longer to depolarize than the right ventricle.

The VAT is measured from the Q wave, or first evidence of ventricular depolarization, to the peak of the R wave (Fig. 11-1).

VAT IN LEFT VENTRICULAR LEADS (V_5 and V_6)

In leads facing the left ventricle, the peak of the R wave occurs in 0.04 sec or less.

VAT IN RIGHT VENTRICULAR LEADS (V_1 and V_2)

In leads facing the right ventricle, the R wave occurs in 0.02 sec or less.

Right bundle branch block (RBBB)

When the impulse is blocked in the right bundle branch, the left ventricle and IV septum are activated normally, and the right ventricle is activated late through the IV septum instead of through the conductive system.

RIGHT VENTRICULAR LEADS (V_1 and V_2) AND THE VAT IN RBBB

Because of the block in conduction through the right bundle branch, the right ventricle will be activated last. This delayed vector will originate in the

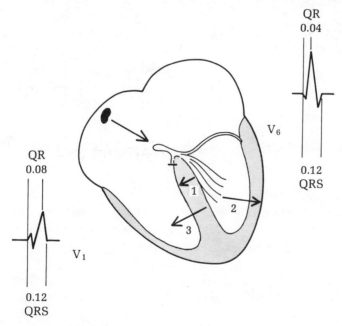

Fig. 11-2. RBBB as reflected in V_1 and V_6.

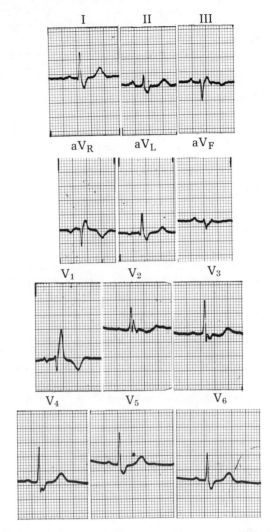

Fig. 11-3. RBBB. Note the late R wave in V_1 and the broad s waves in leads I and V_6, all reflective of late right ventricular activation.

unaffected left side and flows into the positive electrode of V_1, causing broad terminal R′ wave. The VAT is markedly delayed (0.08 sec), as shown i Fig. 11-2. Note that normal septal activation is reflected by the initial little wave. The S wave reflects normal left ventricular activation and the R′ wav late right ventricular activation. The S wave amplitude is usually markedl reduced in RBBB because of the unopposed left-to-right activation of the I septum. Normally the septum is activated mainly from left to right, wit some opposing currents coming from the RBB toward the left. Without the

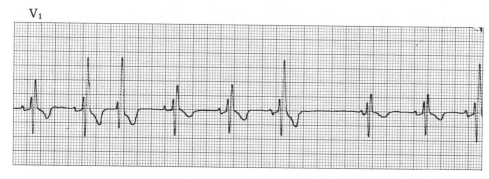

Fig. 11-4. Complete and incomplete right bundle branch block.

opposing forces the net strength of septal activation toward the right is greater. Thus some of the leftward free wall forces are cancelled out, producing a smaller S wave.

EFT VENTRICULAR LEADS (V_5 and V_6) AND THE AT IN RBBB

Since the left ventricle is activated normally, the leads facing this ventricle have a normal VAT (R wave peak) (Fig. 11-2).

RS COMPLEX IN RBBB

The terminal deflection of the QRS complex is the clue to the diagnosis of RBBB. The abnormal, late depolarization of the right ventricle is reflected in this final deflection, which is best seen in V_1 as an R' wave and leads I and V_6 as a broad S wave. The following main ECG features are seen in Fig. 11-3:

1. Prolonged QRS duration (0.11 sec or more)
2. Triphasic complex in V_1 (rSR')
3. T wave changes
4. Peak of R wave (VAT) markedly delayed in right ventricular leads (V_1) and normal in left ventricular leads (V_6)
5. Broad S wave in leads I, aV_L, and V_6

ncomplete RBBB

If the right bundle branch is only partially blocked, the impulse enters the right ventricle through the normal His-Purkinje pathway. However, it is delayed at the site of the block, causing late activation of the right ventricle. This late right ventricular vector is also seen in complete RBBB. Therefore the components of the ventricular complex are the same. The QRS interval, however, is less than 0.11 sec.

Complete and incomplete RBBB are seen in the same tracing in Fig. 11-4.

Left bundle branch block (LBBB)

When the impulse is blocked in the left bundle branch, the IV septal and left ventricular forces are both abnormal. The septum is activated from right to left, and the left ventricle is activated late by right ventricular and septal forces.

RIGHT VENTRICULAR LEADS (V_1 AND V_2) AND THE VAT IN LBBB

The right ventricle is activated normally. Therefore leads facing this ventricle have a normal VAT (0.02 sec), as shown in Fig. 11-5, *A*.

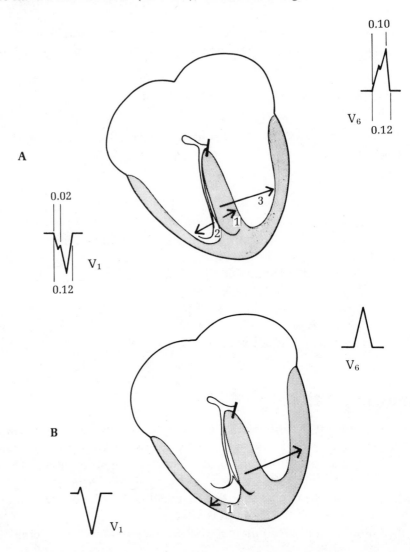

Fig. 11-5. A, LBBB without an r wave in V_1. **B,** LBBB with an r wave in V_1.

EFT VENTRICULAR LEADS (V₅ AND V₆) AND THE
AT IN LBBB

Since the impulse is blocked in the left bundle branch, the left ventricle will be activated late by a vector from the I-V septum instead of via the accelerated pathway of the Purkinje network. Leads facing the left ventricle will therefore have a delayed VAT (more than 0.06 second), as shown in Fig. 11-5, *A*.

RS COMPLEX IN LBBB

The terminal deflection of the QRS complex that reflects the late depolarization of the left ventricle is the clue to diagnosis. Following are the main ECG features:

1. Prolonged QRS interval (0.12 sec or more)
2. Notched deflections in V₆ ("M" slurred complex)
3. T wave changes
4. Peak of R wave (VAT) markedly delayed in left ventricular leads (V₆) and normal in right ventricular leads (V₁)
5. Absent q waves in leads I, aV$_L$, and V₆

The initial forces in LBBB depend on which terminal branch of the RBB is activated first. It will be remembered that there are two main terminal branches to the right bundle. One goes to the IV septum and the other to the anterior papillary muscle. If the septal branch is activated first, the initial forces are septal from right to left, causing the initial deflection in V₁ to be negative. However, if the anterior papillary branch is activated first, the initial forces are directed anteriorly and to the right, causing the initial deflection to be a narrow r wave. These two possibilities are illustrated in Figs. 11-5 to 11-7.

ncomplete LBBB

Partial blockage of the left bundle branch delays the transmission of the impulse through the bundle. The right ventricle is depolarized first with a right-to-left current across the IV septum. The QRS interval is less than 0.12 sec. The diagnosis is therefore made because of the initial right ventricular forces that are the same as those seen in complete LBBB.

The differential diagnosis is sometimes difficult, since the QRS resembles that seen in left ventricular hypertrophy.

Hemiblock

The three main terminal fascicles (bundles) of the intraventricular conduction system are the right bundle branch and the anterior and posterior divisions of the left bundle branch (Fig. 11-8).

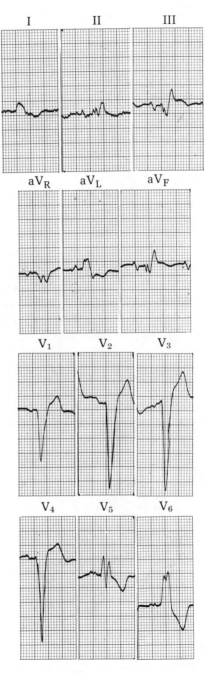

Fig. 11-6. LBBB. Note the delayed VAT in V_6, indicating late activation of the left ventricle, and the absence of q waves in I and V_6, reflective of abnormal septal activation.

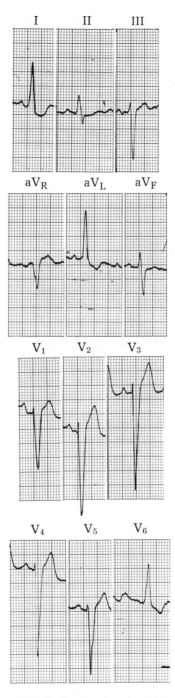

Fig. 11-7. LBBB. Note the r wave in V_1, indicating that the right ventricle was initially activated through the Purkinje fibers in the right ventricular wall.

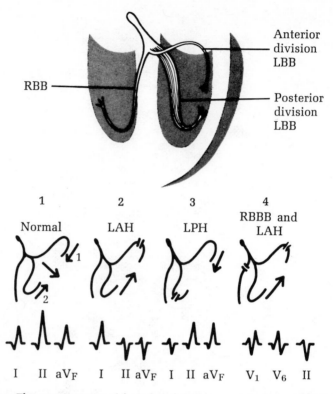

Fig. 11-8. Three main terminal fascicles of the intraventricular conductive system.

When conduction is blocked in either fascicle of the left bundle branch, the condition is referred to as hemiblock: left anterior hemiblock (LAH) or left posterior hemiblock (LPH).

Conduction may be permanently or only intermittently interrupted in one (unifascicular block), two (bifascicular block), or all three (trifascicular block) fascicles. Frequently complete AV block is preceded by the presence of RBBB plus LAH. The anterior division of the left bundle branch has the same anatomical origin as does the right bundle branch, as well as the same blood supply (left coronary artery) (Fig. 11-8). Thus a small lesion may injure both these fascicles.

LEFT ANTERIOR HEMIBLOCK (LAH)

The main blood supply to the anterior division of the left bundle branch comes from the left coronary artery; hence LAH is often seen in anterolateral and anteroseptal myocardial infarction. Because the initial vectors are inferior and to the right (depolarization of the septum), there is a small r wave in leads II, III, and aV$_F$ and a small q wave in lead I. Because the left ventricle is activated through the posterior division of the left bundle branch (Fig. 11-

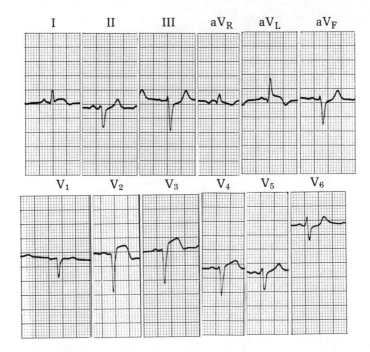

Fig. 11-9. Left anterior hemiblock. Note the mainly positive deflection in I and the negative deflections in II, III, and aV$_F$. The small r waves in the inferior leads and the q wave in lead I differentiate this from inferior wall myocardial infarction.

8), there is a marked left axis deviation (-60 degrees or greater). This is reflected in lead I by a qR and in leads II, III, and aV$_F$ by an rS complex. Fig. 11-9 illustrates LAH.

LEFT ANTERIOR HEMIBLOCK (LAH) AND RBBB

If RBBB is accompanied by a left axis deviation (-60 degrees or greater), LAH is suspected to coexist (Fig. 11-10).

The initial ventricular forces are caused by the hemiblock and determine the direction of the mean QRS axis. The terminal forces are caused by the RBBB. The initial forces cause, as in pure LAH, a small r wave in leads II and aV$_F$, a small q wave in lead I, and S waves in leads II, III, and aV$_F$.

The late activation of the right ventricle due to the RBBB is best seen in lead V$_1$, which has a broad terminal R wave.

LEFT POSTERIOR HEMIBLOCK (LPH) AND RBBB

Block of the posterior division of the left bundle branch is uncommon; because of its breadth, length, position, and dual blood supply (right and left coronary arteries), it is less vulnerable. LPH is almost always associated with RBBB. The ECG manifests a right axis deviation of $+120$ degrees.

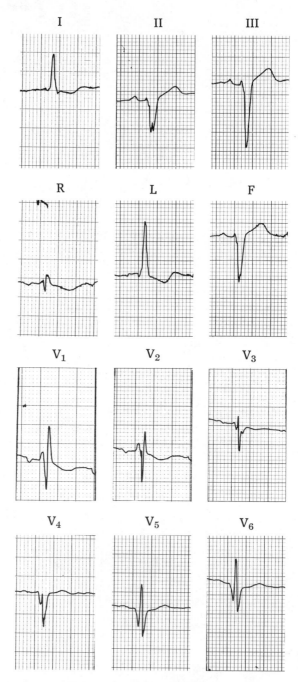

Fig. 11-10. Bifascicular block (RBBB and LAH).

The initial ventricular forces are caused by the LPH and determine the direction of the mean QRS axis. The terminal forces are caused by the RBBB.

Initially the left ventricle is activated through the anterior division of the left bundle branch, causing a small q wave in leads II and aV$_F$ and a small r wave in lead I. Because the posterior wall of the left ventricle and the right ventricular wall are on the same plane, delayed activation of the posterior wall of the left ventricle (LPH) and the late activation of the right ventricle (RBBB) cause an S wave in lead I and R waves in leads II and aV$_F$. Fig. 11-11 reflects LPH and RBBB.

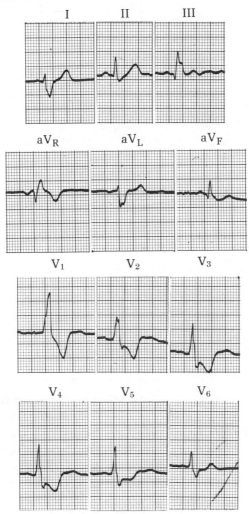

Fig. 11-11. Bifascicular block (RBBB and LPH). Note that lead I is mainly negative, and II and aV$_F$ mainly positive (right axis deviation).

Monitoring procedure in acute anteroseptal myocardial infarction

The anterior wall of the heart and the IV septum receive their blood sup ply from the anterior descending left coronary artery. This artery also sup plies all the bundle branches, being the sole blood supply for the RBB and the anterior division of the LBB. Therefore the conduction problems of a patient with acute anteroseptal myocardial infarction will most probably be at the level of the bundle branches. If there is RBBB, the anterior fascicle is threatened and vice versa. If both RBBB and LAH exist, block of the posterior fascicle would result in complete block and an idioventricular rate incompatible with life. The posterior fascicle is the least threatened because of its dual blood supply and its anatomical structure and position.

In order to be in touch with the conductive system of the patient having acute anteroseptal myocardial infarction, the following monitoring procedure should be observed:

1. With RBBB and a normal axis, monitor on lead II for left axis deviation, with an occasional look at lead I for right axis deviation.
2. When only LAH is present, monitor on V_1 or MCL_1 for RBBB.
3. When the conductive system is intact, monitor on lead II for left axis deviation and/or broadening of the QRS, with an occasional look at lead I for right axis deviation.
4. When both RBBB and LAH are present, monitor on the lead in which the P-R interval is most easily seen. A lengthening of the P-R would indicate further block, perhaps in the posterior fascicle.
5. When there is a differential diagnosis between ventricular ectopy and aberration, V_1 (or MCL_1) and V_6 (or MCL_6) are the leads in which morphology is helpful. Aberrant ventricular conduction is discussed in Chapter 12.

Rationale
RBBB AND A NORMAL AXIS

When the patient with anteroseptal myocardial infarction has RBBB, there is a danger of LAH, since both fascicles share the same blood supply. Note that in Fig. 11-12, *A*, the patient has RBBB with a normal axis. A little later, in Fig. 11-12, *B*, there is both RBBB and LAH. Note that the only lead in which this change is apparent is in lead II. The axis shift is not seen in V_1 or MCL_1, nor is it detected in leads I or III because lead I is normally positive and lead III may normally be negative. Thus your monitoring lead for a patient with acute anteroseptal myocardial infarction and RBBB is lead II. You should also occasionally evaluate lead I for LPH, which is reflected by a right axis deviation. Note that in Fig. 11-13 the axis has shifted from normal to

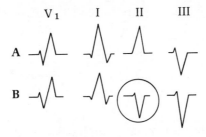

Fig. 11-12. A, Patient has RBBB and a normal axis. A little later, **B,** left anterior hemiblock has complicated the picture. Note that the only lead in which this is detected is lead II.

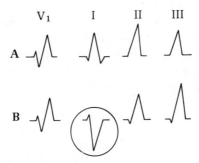

Fig. 11-13. A, Patient has RBBB and a normal axis. A little later, **B,** left posterior hemiblock has complicated the picture. Note that the only lead in which this is detected is lead I.

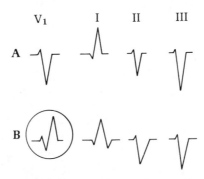

Fig. 11-14. A, Patient has left anterior hemiblock reflected by a left axis deviation. **B,** RBBB has complicated the picture. Note that the lead in which this is best detected is lead V_1 (or MCL_1).

right and that lead I is the only lead to reflect this change because leads II and III may normally be upright.

LEFT AXIS DEVIATION WITHOUT RBBB

If the patient has only LAH, then one must monitor in a lead in which RBBB is most easily detected. Note that in Fig. 11-14, *A*, the patient has LAH. Later in Fig. 11-14, *B*, there is also RBBB. In the limb leads the QRS broad-

ens and an S wave appears in lead I, but the change that one would notic
most easily on the monitor is clearly in V_1 or MCl_1. Thus your monitorin
lead for a patient with acute anteroseptal myocardial infarction and LAH i
V_1 or MCL_1.

Summary

Right and left bundle branch blocks are distinctive intraventricular con
duction defects. The most significant ECG feature of each is the late activa
tion of the affected ventricle. This is most easily recognized in the right and
left precordial leads.

The conductive system of the heart is trifascicular in structure. The lef
bundle branch has two divisions (anterior and posterior). A block of the an
terior division is termed *left anterior hemiblock* and a block of the posterior
division is termed *left posterior hemiblock*. LAH and RBBB often coexist and
as a precursor of symptomatic AV block take on important diagnosti
significance.

CHAPTER 12

Aberrant ventricular conduction

Aberrant means straying from the right way or wandering. In electro-cardiography the term is used to indicate that although an impulse may have entered the ventricle in the normal way through the AV node and bundle of His, its pathway within the ventricles is errant. The term applies only to the transient conduction defect.

Aberrant ventricular conduction occurs most often when, because of (1) rapid rates, (2) very premature atrial contractions, and/or (3) changes in cycle length, the His-Purkinje system is not completely repolarized and is therefore functionally unable to conduct normally. In addition to incomplete repolarization, causes of aberrancy may also be a reduction in the membrane potential and/or in the rate of rise of phase 0 of the action potential (membrane responsiveness).

Because the right bundle branch repolarizes slightly later than the left bundle branch, it is most susceptible to block. This is the pattern (RBBB) most often assumed by the aberrant ventricular impulse.

Differentiation between aberrant ventricular conduction and ectopic ventricular complexes on the basis of morphology

Aberrant ventricular conduction takes the form of RBBB 80% of the time. The rest of the time it is LBBB or hemiblock. It is therefore important to know the morphology of BBB.

RBBB ABERRATION VERSUS LEFT VENTRICULAR ECTOPY

Since left ventricular ectopic beats produce a mainly positive deflection in V_1 and RBBB does also, the main morphological differentiation is between these two mechanisms, as illustrated in Fig. 12-1. Most of the time, RBBB aberration is reflected in V_1 and V_6 by its typical triphasic pattern, that is, an rSR' in V_1 and a qRs in V_6.

In left ventricular ectopy the mainly positive deflection in V_1 often has two peaks, with the *initial* peak being taller. In V_6 helpful clues to ventricular ectopy are either a QS or an rS pattern. All these complexes are illustrated in Fig. 12-1.

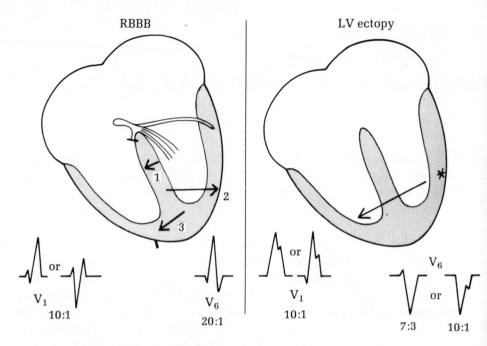

Fig. 12-1. Morphological differentiation between RBBB and left ventricular ectopy.

LBBB ABERRATION VERSUS RIGHT VENTRICULAR ECTOPY

When aberration takes the form of LBBB, it produces a mainly negative deflection in V_1 and so does right ventricular ectopy. In a small percentage of cases a differentiation can be made between the two mechanisms if a little r wave is present in V_1. In the case of LBBB such an r wave would be narrow, whereas in right ventricular ectopy it may be broad (greater than 0.03 sec).

ADDITIONAL HELPFUL CLUES

Ventricular tachycardia is usually regular and may have concordant patterns in the precordial leads. The axis in ventricular tachycardia is commonly either to the left or in no-man's-land (± 180 to -90 degrees).

For a decade these morphological clues have been offered by Marriott.[1-3] They have been developed through observation and deductive reasoning and without invasive studies. Recently the Wellens group[4] in the Netherlands has performed invasive cardiac studies on 122 patients and was able to study 140 episodes of tachycardia. Their findings confirm those of Marriott and have also yielded additional clues: (1) ventricular tachycardia usually has a QRS wider than 0.14 sec; (2) supraventricular tachycardia usually has a narrower QRS of only 0.12 sec (53 out of 63 cases); and (3) in a small

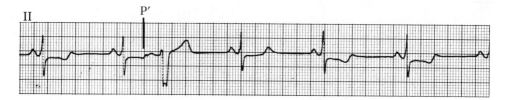

Fig. 12-2. Premature atrial complex (PAC) with AVC.

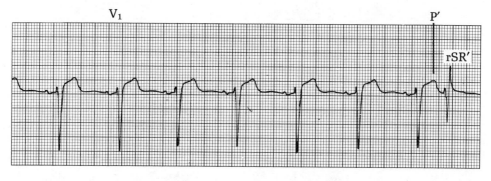

Fig. 12-3. RBBB aberration following a PAC.

percentage of cases (8%)[4] ventricular tachycardia has a wide QR in leads I and/or V_6.

Premature atrial complexes (PACs) and aberrant ventricular conduction (AVC)

AVC following a PAC is commonly mistaken for a premature ventricular complex (PVC), especially when the P' wave is hidden in the preceding T wave. A less than full compensatory pause should alert you to examine the preceding T wave more carefully for signs of a premature atrial beat. Occasionally, however, a full compensatory pause follows the PAC because an ectopic stimulus in the atria may suppress the sinus node pacemaker. Suppression of the sinus node may delay the next impulse long enough for it to occur at the normal time.

The premature complex shown in Fig. 12-2 seems, at a glance, to be a PVC. However, there is not a full compensatory pause, and after close examination a P' wave can be seen on the preceding T wave. This is a PAC with AVC.

At a rate of 48 this tracing also represents sinus bradycardia. When the ventricular rate decreases, the time taken for the repolarization process lengthens. It is therefore more likely that a premature atrial stimulus will

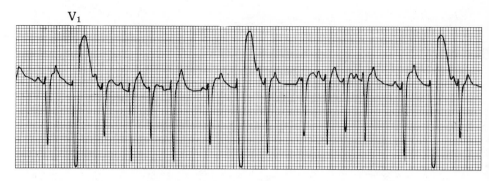

Fig. 12-4. Chaotic atrial tachycardia with LBBB aberration.

meet with refractory tissue when the dominant rate is slow. The coupling interval is of course also a factor. The closer the PAC is to the preceding ventricular complex, the more inevitable is aberration. Both a lengthened action potential due to bradycardia and a short coupling interval are causative factors in the AVC shown in Fig. 12-2.

In V_1 aberrant ventricular conduction is more easily recognized because it commonly takes the form of RBBB. Fig. 12-3 illustrates a PAC conducted with RBBB aberrancy. The typical rSR' pattern is noted in the last complex, and a P' wave can be presumed to be the cause of the slightly distorted T wave preceding the aberrant complex.

The three broad-looking complexes in the chaotic atrial tachycardia seen in Fig. 12-4 represent LBBB aberrancy. P' waves are evident in the T wave preceding the aberrant complex. Note that the r wave of the aberrant complex is narrow. The differential diagnosis would be between LBBB aberrancy and right ventricular ectopy. In the latter the r wave would more likely be broad. It is also noted in this tracing that both a short and then a long cycle precede the aberrant beat. The long cycle would cause the following beat to have a longer refractory period. Thus it is that the PAC has a greater chance of being conducted aberrantly.

ATRIAL FIBRILLATION AND AVC

When P waves are present, one can often make the diagnosis of aberrancy because of a visible P' wave. In atrial fibrillation no such clue is available and one is left only with the morphological clues. To give further credence to these clues, Vera et al.,[5] using His bundle electrography, analyzed abnormal QRS complexes in 1100 patients with chronic atrial fibrillation. Of these, 750 were found to be ventricular ectopic beats, and 350 were aberrantly conducted supraventricular beats. V_1 (or MCL_1) was found to be the single most helpful lead in differentiating ectopy from aberrancy. In this lead an rSR' pattern was 24:1 in favor of aberrancy, and a qR or monophasic R pattern was 9:1 in favor of ectopy.

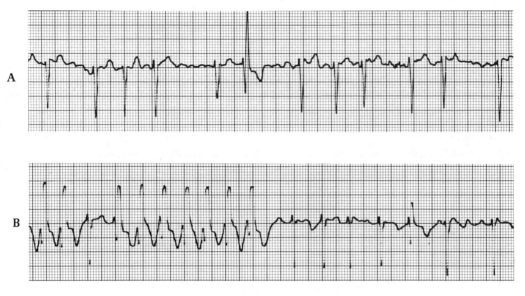

Fig. 12-5. Atrial fibrillation with RBBB aberration.

It was also found that fixed or variable coupling intervals, bigeminal rhythms, long-short cycle (Ashman's phenomenon), and a long pause following the anomalous beat were of little diagnostic value. When a bizarre QRS axis, concordancy of the precordial leads, or R-on-T phenomenon were encountered, the anomalous beat was found to be ectopic.

Fig. 12-5, *A*, illustrates RBBB aberration in atrial fibrillation. Fig. 12-5, *B*, is from the same patient and illustrates the same rSR' pattern as a clue to the supraventricular origin of the tachycardia.

In Fig. 12-6 the broad complexes have a wide R wave in V_1. This favors the diagnosis of right ventricular ectopy over LBBB aberration. Compare these ectopic complexes with the aberrant complexes in Fig. 12-4.

ATRIAL FLUTTER AND AVC

AVC is evident in the tracing of atrial flutter seen in Fig. 12-7. The first aberrant complex follows a short cycle that is preceded by a longer cycle, thus lengthening the refractory period of the beat following the pause and making aberration more probable in the next complex. All aberrant beats in this tracing take the form of RBBB, with the last two complexes reflecting incomplete and then complete RBBB aberration.

SUPRAVENTRICULAR TACHYCARDIA AND AVC

When the ventricular rate suddenly becomes more rapid, the repolarization time does not change suddenly. Rather, there is a gradual adjustment. The suddenly accelerated stimulus in some cases meets with incompletely re-

V₁

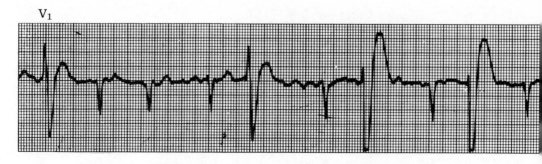

Fig. 12-6. Atrial fibrillation and ventricular ectopic beats.

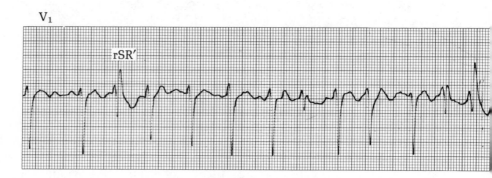

Fig. 12-7. Atrial flutter with RBBB aberration.

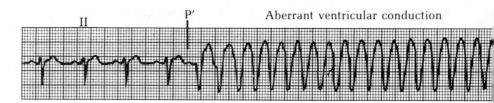

Fig. 12-8. Onset of supraventricular tachycardia with AVC.

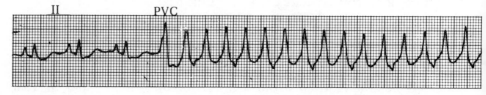

Fig. 12-9. Onset of ventricular tachycardia.

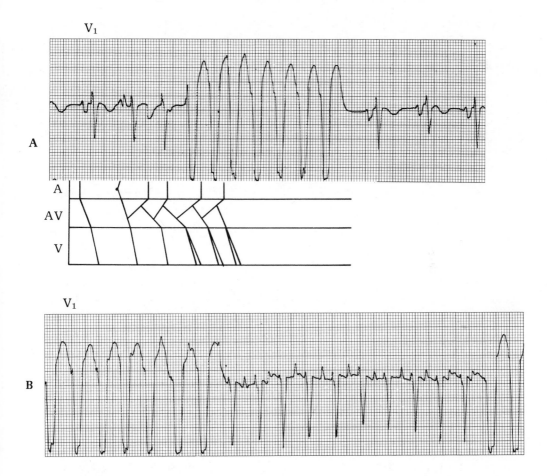

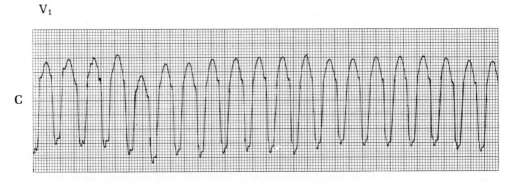

Fig. 12-10. Three tracings from the same patient. **A,** PAC can be seen to initiate a reciprocating tachycardia with aberrant ventricular conduction (LBBB). **B,** The aberrancy is intermittent and the P′ waves are clearly seen. **C,** Neither the onset nor the P′ waves are seen, making it almost impossible to differentiate between AVC and ventricular ectopy.

polarized tissue in the bundle branches and results in aberrant ventricular complexes. A classic example of this is shown in Fig. 12-8.

OTHER CLUES

A differential diagnosis between aberration and ectopy can more easily be made if the following are seen: the onset of the tachycardia, isolated extrasystoles, visible P waves, and Dressler beats, as well as right bundle branch block (RBBB) pattern in the aberrant complex.

Onset of the tachycardia

A premature P' wave is often seen preceding a supraventricular tachycardia (Fig. 12-8). A premature ventricular beat is seen initiating a ventricular tachycardia. Such is the case in Fig. 12-9, where the ventricular tachycardia is accompanied by retrograde conduction to the atria with each alternate beat (2:1 retrograde conduction).

In Fig. 12-10, A, tachycardia can be seen to have been initiated by a PAC. A reciprocating rhythm with LBBB aberration results. Note the narrow r wave of the first aberrant beat. This is a distinguishing feature between LBBB and right ventricular ectopy. In Fig. 12-10, B, intermittent normal intraventricular conduction is seen. Fig. 12-10, C, is from the same patient. Without the tracings preceding, it would have been difficult to differentiate between aberration and ectopy on the basis of information from the surface ECG alone.

Isolated extrasystoles

A diagnosis of supraventricular tachycardia with AVC would be reasonably certain if an AVC complex of the same contour as the tachycardia were

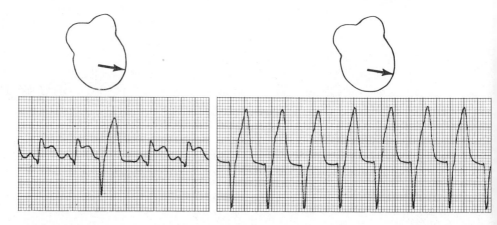

12-11. Isolated premature ventricular contraction (PVC) of the same morphology as that of the ventricular tachycardia.

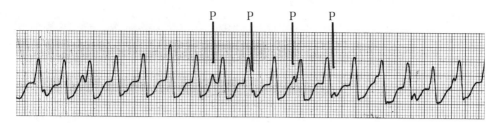

Fig. 12-12. Sign of dissociation in ventricular tachycardia.

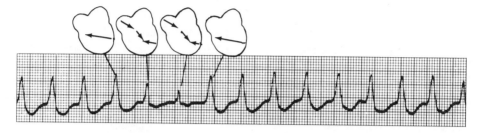

Fig. 12-13. Ventricular tachycardia with Dressler beats (ventricular fusion).

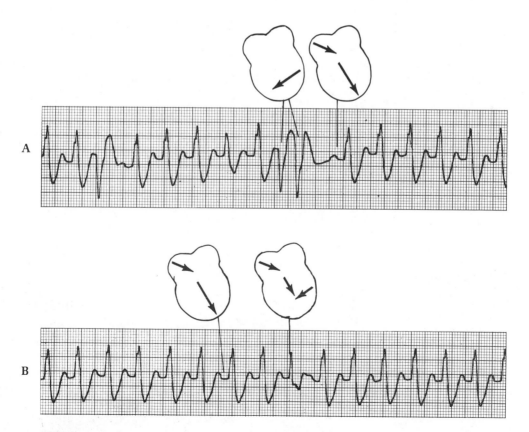

A

B

Fig. 12-14. A, Supraventricular tachycardia with PVCs. **B,** Same patient. Supraventricular tachycardia with a ventricular fusion beat, which resembles a Dressler beat.

seen in a preceding isolated complex. By the same token, a diagnosis of ventricular tachycardia would be certain if an isolated PVC of the same contour as the tachycardia were seen in a previous tracing. For example, a previous tracing of the patient in Fig. 12-11 shows an isolated PVC of the same morphology as that of the tachycardia.

Visible P waves

Independent P waves that are dissociated from ventricular activity are supportive but not conclusive evidence of ventricular tachycardia (Fig. 12-12).

Conversely, if a P wave is seen in relation to each anomalous complex, a diagnosis of supraventricular tachycardia cannot always be made, since this relationship may also be seen in ventricular tachycardia with 1 : 1 retrograde conduction. However, if the P' wave is upright in lead II, one would be safe in assuming that the pacemaker was in the atrium and that impulses were being conducted to the ventricle.

Dressler beats

Narrower beats of lesser amplitude, such as those seen in Fig. 12-13, are caused by ventricular fusion and when seen in ventricular tachycardia are termed Dressler beats.

Dressler beats are suggestive of, but not diagnostic of, ventricular tachycardia. They are seldom seen when the rate is over 150.

In Fig. 12-14, *B*, the narrower complex that interrupts the series of broad, tall ventricular complexes is a ventricular fusion beat. In this case, however, it is caused by a ventricular ectopic vector fusing with a sinus-conducted impulse. In the first tracing (Fig. 12-14, *A*) the complexes from both foci can be seen. The coupled PVCs are followed by a compensatory pause that allows one to see the sinus P wave and its ventricular response. This ventricular response manifests the same QRS contour as is seen in the tachycardia. Thus there is no doubt that the tachycardia is supraventricular (sinus) in origin.

Summary

Ventricular aberration occurs if the ventricle is still partially refractory at the time of the next stimulus. The term *AVC* is reserved for the occasional errant pathway that a supraventricular stimulus takes through the ventricle and applies only to a transient conduction defect (functional BBB).

PACs with AVC are frequently misdiagnosed as PVCs. Look for the premature P' wave hidden in the T. Measure the compensatory pause. Differentiating between supraventricular tachycardia and ventricular tachycardia is often impossible with the ECG alone. Following are a few clues[1-5]:

Aberration	Ectopy
1. rSR′ in V_1	1. When there are two positive peaks in V_1, initial one is usually taller.
2. qRs in V_6	2. QS or rS in V_6
3. When there is an rS in V_1, the r is narrow.	3. When there is an rS in V_1, the r is broad (>0.03 sec).
4. QRS narrow (0.12 sec) (53 out of 63)	4. QRS wider than 0.14 sec
	5. Wide QR in leads I and/or V_6 (6 out of 70)
	6. Axis: left or in no-man's-land
	7. Concordant patterns in precordial leads

References

1. Marriott, H. J. L.: Differential diagnosis of supraventricular and ventricular tachycardia, Geriatrics **25**:91, 1970.
2. Marriott, H. J. L.: Practical electrocardiography, ed. 6, Baltimore, 1977, The Williams & Wilkins Co.
3. Marriott, H. J. L.: Workshop in electrocardiography, Oldsmar, Fla., 1972, Tampa Tracings.
4. Wellens, H. J. J., Bär, F. W. H. M., and Lie, K. I.: The value of the electrocardiogram in the differential diagnosis of a tachycardia with a widened QRS complex, Am. J. Med. **64**:27, 1978.
5. Vera, Z., Cheng, T. O., Ertem, G., Shoaleh-var, M., Wickramasekaran, R., and Wadhwa, K.: His bundle electrography for evaluation of criteria in differentiating ventricular ectopy from aberrancy in atrial fibrillation, Circulation **45**(supp. 2):355, 1972.

CHAPTER 13

Preexcitation syndrome

Definition

Preexcitation exists when all or part of the ventricular muscle is activated by an atrial impulse earlier than would occur if activation had proceeded normally through the AV node and bundle of His.[1] Such a syndrome is of interest because it often results in debilitating reentrant tachycardia and/or atrial fibrillation that may lead to very high ventricular rates. Sudden death in these patients may be the result of ventricular fibrillation[2] if atrial fibrillation is accompanied by a short refractory period in the accessory pathway.

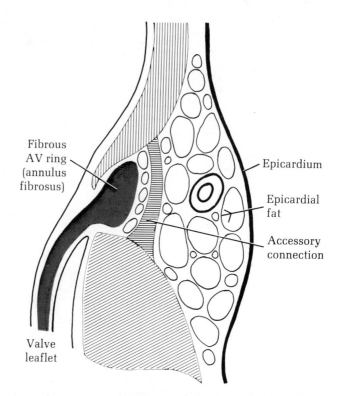

Fig. 13-1. Diagrammatic representation of a left-sided accessory atrioventricular connection. Note that the connection skirts through the epicardial fat, being outside the AV fibrous ring. (From Becker, A. E., Anderson, R. H., Durrer, D., and Wellens, H. J. J.: Circulation **57**:870, 1978. By permission of the American Heart Association, Inc.)

Embryology

In the embryo the myocardium of the atria is continuous with that of the ventricles until eventually connective tissue and then fibrous tissue separate atria from ventricles. At the connective tissue stage some muscular connections still persist and are normally severed by the development of a fibrous band (AV ring), leaving only one muscular tract, the bundle of His, connecting atria, and ventricles.

Some authorities[3,4] have postulated that in patients with preexcitation one or more of these muscular connections may fail to be severed by the development of the fibrous tissue around the AV ring.

Others[5] have not found such proof of the faulty embryological development described but have found in four left-sided connections that the accessory bundle was separate from an intact AV ring. Fig. 13-1 illustrates these recent findings.

Such anomalous *tracts* (inserting into conductive tissue) or *connections* (inserting into myocardium)[6] may be single or multiple,[7] active or inactive,[8] and may possess the capability of conducting both anterogradely and retrogradely. In a significant number of individuals with preexcitation syndrome the accessory pathway conducts only retrogradely (concealed WPW syndrome).[9-11]

Classification of preexcitation syndrome

There are three classifications of preexcitation syndrome, according to where the accessory pathway has its origin and insertion.

1. If an extra muscle bundle forms a connection between atria and ventricle outside the conductive system, it is called the *Wolff-Parkinson-White syndrome.*
2. If a muscle tract bypasses the AV node and inserts into the bundle of His, it is referred to as the *short P-R syndrome.*
3. There may be fasciculoventricular and/or nodoventricular connections that are sometimes called *Mahaim fibers.*

Wolff-Parkinson-White (WPW) syndrome: an accessory AV connection
HISTORICAL BACKGROUND

In 1930 Wolff, Parkinson, and White[12] described bundle-branch block with short P-R interval in healthy young people prone to paroxysmal tachycardia. This description was made without reference to AV bypass tracts. Connections between the atria and ventricles had, however, been described by Kent[13] as early as 1893 and before that by Paladino[14] in 1876. These AV connections have been called the *bundles of Kent* and are diagrammatically

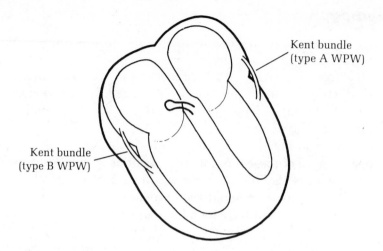

Fig. 13-2. Diagrammatic representation of the bundles of Kent responsible for types A and B WPW syndrome.

Table 1. Shortest normal P-R and longest normal QRS according to age*

Age	P-R (sec)	QRS (sec)
0 to 6 mo	0.08	0.06
6 mo to 3 yr	0.08	0.08
3 to 5 yr	0.10	0.08
5 to 16 yr	0.10	0.09
Older than 16 yr	0.12	0.10

*Modified from Ferrer, M. I.: Electrocardiographic notebook, ed. 4, Mount Kisco, N.Y., 1973, Futura Publishing Co.

illustrated in Fig. 13-2. It was not until 1932 and 1933[15,16] that the concept of AV bypass tracts capable of transmitting impulses from atria to ventricles ahead of the normal sequence was suggested. By 1943 and 1944[17,18] the ECG criteria for WPW syndrome were linked with postmortem histological confirmation of the presence of AV bypass tracts on the right and left sides of the heart.

ECG CRITERIA FOR WPW SYNDROME

The three classical ECG features of WPW syndrome are (1) a short P-R interval (<0.12 sec), (2) a broad QRS complex (>0.10 sec) and (3) a delta wave. This syndrome is the most common of the preexcitation syndromes.[19-21]

The P/R interval. Note in Fig. 13-2 that the two bundles of Kent are totally separate from the normal AV conduction system. Thus, impulses conducted over either Kent bundle would not experience the normal delay accomplished by the AV node. The P-R interval would, therefore, usually be

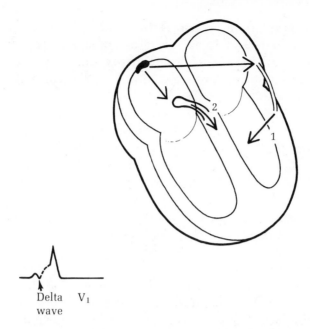

Delta   V₁
wave

Fig. 13-3. Delta wave in type A WPW syndrome. Note that this low-frequency component of the QRS complex is the result of early ventricular activation and slow conduction outside the interventricular conductive system. Note also that the delta force usually collides with the electrical currents proceeding normally through the AV junction. Thus the QRS is generally a fusion beat.

shortened. (The shortest normal P-R interval according to age is displayed in Table 1.) This shortening of the P-R interval will take place as long as conduction time through the atria and across the accessory pathway is shorter than if it had traveled its normal AV route. However, if the accessory pathway is situated on the opposite side of the heart from the sinus node, the sinus impulse may reach the ventricles simultaneously through the normal AV junctional pathway and through the accessory pathway. In such a case the P-R interval would be normal. Other contributing factors to a normal P-R interval in WPW syndrome are (1) delayed intra-atrial conduction time, (2) delayed conduction velocity in the accessory pathway, and/or (3) excessive length of the accessory pathway.

The QRS complex and the delta wave. The term *degree of preexcitation* refers to the degree of ventricular activation by way of the accessory pathway. This determines the width of the QRS complex and is itself determined by how quickly the sinus impulse passes through the atria and across the accessory pathway. The ventricles may be totally activated through the accessory pathway (maximum preexcitation), or the impulse may arrive in the ventricles across the accessory pathway only slightly before it arrives by way of the AV junction (minimum preexcitation). Any degree of preexcitation in between these two extremes is possible. It is also possible for the sinus impulse to arrive in the ventricles simultaneously through both the normal and abnormal pathways. In such a case, although there is no preexcitation, the consequences of WPW syndrome (paroxysmal supraventricular tachycardia and/or atrial fibrillation) would still exist for that patient.[22]

When the sinus impulse arrives in the ventricles first through the accessory pathway, it begins its ventricular conduction outside the conductive system, resulting in an initial slurring of the QRS complex called a *delta wave*. It is the delta wave that causes the widening of the QRS complex. This is diagrammatically illustrated in Fig. 13-3. Note in this illustration that the excitation wave also enters through the AV node and bundle of His, causing a ventricular fusion complex.[23,24]

If the sinus impulse arrives in the ventricles simultaneously through both pathways, there is of course no delta wave, and the P-R interval is normal. However, because of the simultaneous activation of the ventricles from two sites (a fusion beat), the following QRS abnormalities may exist: (1) abnormal Q waves, (2) slurring of the ascending limb of the R wave, (3) increased voltage of the QRS complex and (4) axis shift. There would then be a differential diagnosis between WPW syndrome and the following: (1) myocardial infarction, (2) other interventricular conduction disturbances, and (3) ventricular hypertrophy.[22]

The T wave. Because ventricular depolarization does not follow a normal sequence, the repolarization process will also be out of sequence, causing T wave changes dependent on the degree and area of preexcitation.[22]

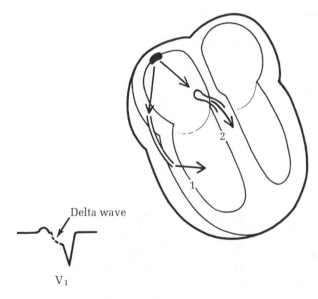

Fig. 13-4. Delta wave in type B WPW syndrome.

Abnormal Q waves. Abnormal Q waves (amplitude of 25% of the succeeding R wave and/or duration of 0.04 sec or greater) are often seen in WPW syndrome. Such Q waves are really negative delta waves and are pointed out in Figs. 13-5 to 13-7.

TYPES A AND B WPW

In 1945[25] WPW syndrome was classified as types A and B according to the polarity of the QRS complex in V_1. When there was an R wave in this lead, it was classified as type A, illustrated in Fig. 13-3. When the complex in V_1 was predominantly negative, it was classified as type B, illustrated in Fig. 13-4. Later it was demonstrated that type B WPW syndrome was caused by a Kent bundle on the right side of the heart and that type A was the result of a Bundle on the left side.[26,27]

It should be noted that this method of determining the location of the bypass tract is oversimplified. QRS configuration can be a guide, however, only

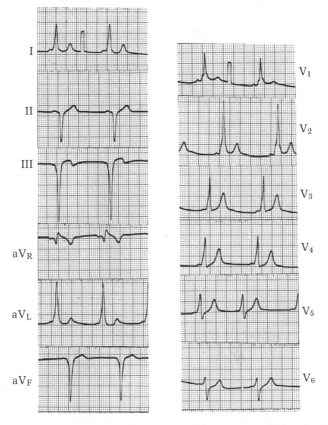

Fig. 13-5. Type A WPW syndrome. Note the positive delta wave in all the chest leads and the negative delta wave in the inferior leads. (Courtesy Dr. Ara G. Tilkian.)

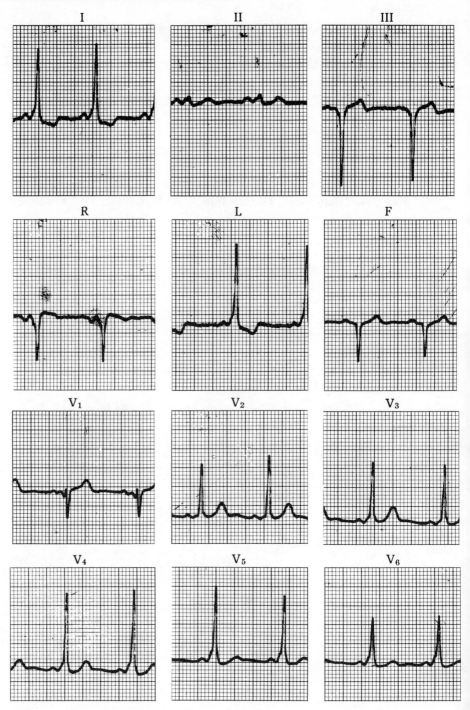

Fig. 13-6. Type B WPW syndrome. Note the QS pattern in V_1 and in leads III and aV_F (F). (From Conover, M. H.: Cardiac arrhythmias: exercises in pattern interpretation, ed. 2, St. Louis, 1978, The C. V. Mosby Co.)

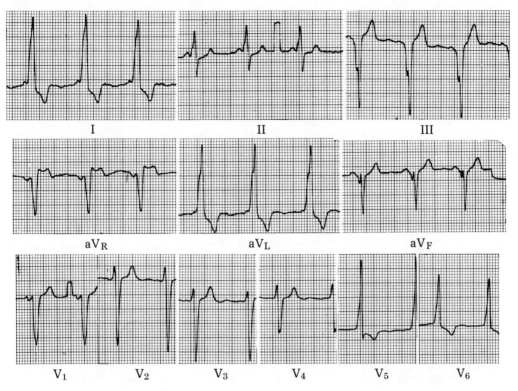

Fig. 13-7. Type B WPW syndrome. Note the rS pattern sometimes seen in V_1 and the QS in leads III and aV_F. (Courtesy Dr. Burton W. Fink.)

if there is maximum preexcitation; that is, only when ventricular activation is mostly over the accessory pathway.[22]

Fig. 13-5 illustrates a 12-lead ECG from a patient with type A WPW syndrome. A positive delta wave is clearly seen in all the chest leads and in leads I and aV_L. Note the pathological Q waves in the inferior leads. They are really negative delta waves, which are often mistaken as an indication of inferior wall myocardial infarction.

Figs. 13-6 and 13-7 illustrate type B WPW. In Fig. 13-6 a negative delta wave is easily seen in V_1. Again there are negative delta waves (Q waves) in the inferior leads masquerading as inferior wall myocardial infarction.

RRHYTHMIAS IN WPW SYNDROME

Patients with WPW syndrome are prone to a circus movement tachycardia, atrial fibrillation, or both.[22]

The circus movement tachycardia mechanism in WPW syndrome is the prototype of reentry. The circuit may be initiated by a critically timed atrial or ventricular extrasystole.[28]

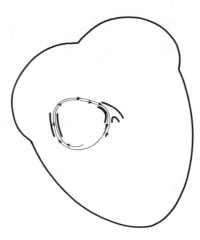

Fig. 13-8. Diagrammatic representation of the circus movement mechanism in the tachycard associated with WPW syndrome.

If a PAC initiates the tachycardia, the current is usually blocked in th accessory pathway, since its refractory period in the anterograde directio usually exceeds that of the AV node. Thus the impulse passes normally dow the AV junction to produce a normal QRS or BBB aberration, then retre gradely up the accessory pathway to activate the atria and back down the A node and bundle of His again. Such a circus movement is diagrammatical illustrated in Fig. 13-8. This mechanism may result in rates of 120 to 23 beats/min.[29] The tachycardia may be electrocardiographically indistinguis able from the reciprocating tachycardia that is confined to the AV node e cept that when an accessory pathway is involved, the P' wave always fo lows the QRS, the P'-R interval being longer than the R-P' interval in mo cases.[22] In AV nodal reentry tachycardia the P' wave is hidden within th QRS complex in more than half the cases (p. 87).

Rarely, the PAC may be conducted anterogradely through the accessor pathway, producing a broad QRS because of maximal preexcitation. It the passes retrogradely through the AV junction. Such a tachycardia would b electrocardiographically indistinguishable from ventricular tachycardia e cept that P' waves always follow the QRS when there is an accessory path way. It may also be indistinguishable from atrial tachycardia or flutter wit 1:1 conduction over the accessory pathway.

When the initiating impulse of the tachycardia is a PVC, the current usu ally passes retrogradely up the accessory pathway, presumably because in retrograde direction the refractory period of the accessory pathway is short than that of the bundle of His–AV node route.[28] Thus following the initiatin PVC, the QRS complexes are normal in configuration or are of BBB aberra tion.

Atrial fibrillation may occur in approximately 11.5% of patients with WPW syndrome.[29] If this is associated with a short refractory period in the accessory pathway, the resulting arrhythmia may be life threatening[24] degenerating into ventricular fibrillation. In fact, the presenting symptom may be ventricular fibrillation.[2]

In some patients the atrial fibrillation may be the result of the reciprocating tachycardia typical of WPW syndrome in that the rapid atrial firing may lead to disorganization of the atrial rhythm.[24,30] Ventricular premature beats conducting retrogradely over the accessory pathway may also initiate the atrial fibrillation.[24]

ONCEALED WPW SYNDROME

In concealed WPW syndrome there is an accessory pathway present that conducts only in a retrograde direction. Thus the ECG of these patients is normal when they are in sinus rhythm.[31] They can therefore be diagnosed only during the tachycardia because the P' wave follows the QRS just as it does in manifest WPW syndrome. Additionally, if the accessory pathway is left sided, there is a negative P' wave in lead I during the tachycardia.

Concealed WPW syndrome should not be confused with the condition in which anterograde conduction over the accessory pathway is simultaneous with conduction over the AV junction. This, too, as stated on p. 157, results in a normal P-R and a narrow QRS complex, yet in this case there is anterograde conduction over the accessory pathway, whereas in concealed WPW there is not.

Because the treatment of patients with concealed WPW differs from that of patients with AV nodal reentrant tachycardia, it is important to make the differential diagnosis. Sung et al.[31] have made the following observations in regard to concealed WPW syndrome:

1. The patient presents with intractable episodes of supraventricular tachycardia.
2. The tachycardia may not be initiated by a PAC or PJC but may have a spontaneous onset following an acceleration of the sinus or atrial rate.
3. If aberrant ventricular conduction develops during the tachycardia, the rate slows down during this period.
4. Associated atrial flutter or fibrillation is present.

IGNS AND SYMPTOMS OF CIRCUS MOVEMENT TACHYCARDIA N WPW SYNDROME

Wellens et al.[22] recently reported on the complaints of patients with proven circus movement tachycardia involving the accessory pathway. Young patients experienced anginal pain when the tachycardia was in excess of 200 beats/min. Almost all patients were aware of the tachycardia, as well as its abrupt beginning and ending. Other symptoms were dyspnea, perspiration, fatigue, anxiety, dizziness, and polyuria.

Short P-R and normal QRS (Lown-Ganong-Levine syndrome): AV nodal bypass

In 1952 Lown, Ganong, and Levine[32] reported the syndrome of short P-R interval, normal QRS complex, and paroxysmal rapid heart action. Anatomical and physiological correlations for this syndrome are controversial concerning whether or not the short P-R and supraventricular tachycardia manifested by these patients are the result of an AV nodal bypass tract,[33] an anatomically small AV node,[34] or of rapidly conducting preferential intranodal fibers.[35]

Wellens and also Josephson and Kastor[35] have reported the tachycardia circuit in these patients to be completely confined to the AV node.

Mahaim fibers: nodoventricular or fasciculoventricular connections

In 1941 Mahaim[36,37] described anomalous connections between the AV node or bundle of His and the ventricle. Fig. 13-9 illustrates a nodoventricular accessory connection. The P-R interval and QRS duration in this case would depend on the origin and insertion of the extra fiber as well as it

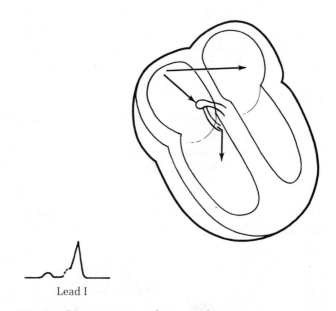

Lead I

Fig. 13-9. Diagrammatic nodoventricular accessory connection.

length. Characteristically there is a small delta wave, a P-R interval that is longer than that of the classical WPW syndrome, and a QRS duration that is increased but not as much as it is in classical WPW.[38]

It should be noted that this type of preexcitation is almost impossible to distinguish on the 12-lead ECG from that of WPW syndrome with minimal preexcitation. Remember that the degree of preexcitation in WPW syndrome is dependent on several factors, as discussed on p. 157. When conduction over the bundle of Kent only slightly precedes that over the AV junction, the P-R is a little longer and the QRS a little shorter. Thus, without electrophysiological studies it is impossible to determine whether it is a Mahaim fiber or a Kent bundle that is responsible for the preexcitation. In fact, it has been shown that more than one accessory pathway can exist[39-41] in the same heart.

Summary

The preexcitation syndrome is said to exist when the ventricle is activated by an atrial impulse earlier than would occur if activation had proceeded normally through the AV node and bundle of His. There are three types of preexcitation:

1. Accessory AV pathway (WPW syndrome), reflected by a short P-R, a broad QRS, and a delta wave
2. AV nodal bypass tract (short P-R, normal QRS syndrome)
3. Mahaim fibers that are either nodoventricular or fasciculoventricular and manifest with (a) a P-R that may be longer than that of the classical WPW but may be normal or shorter than normal, (b) a QRS shorter than that of the classical WPW but longer than normal and (c) a small delta wave

References

1. Durrer, D.: Electrical aspects of human cardiac activity: a clinical-physiological approach to excitation and stimulation, Cardiovasc. Res. **2**:1, 1968.
2. Bashore, T. M., Sellers, T. D., Gallagher, J. J., and Wallace, A. G.: Ventricular fibrillation in the Wolff-Parkinson-White syndrome, Circulation **53**(supp. 2):187, 1976.
3. Ferrer, M. I.: Preexcitation. Am. J. Med. **62**:715, 1977.
4. Verduyn-Lunel, A. A.: Significance of annulus fibrosus of heart in relation to AV conduction and ventricular activation in cases of Wolff-Parkinson-White syndrome, Br. Heart J. **34**:1263, 1972.
5. Becker, A. E., Anderson, R. H., Durrer, D., and Wellens, H. J. J.: The anatomical substrates of Wolff-Parkinson-White syndrome: a clinicopathologic correlation in seven patients, Circulation **57**:870, 1978.
6. Anderson, R. H., Becker, A. E., Brechenmacher, C., et al.: Ventricular preexcitation: a proposed nomenclature for its substrates, Eur. J. Cardiol. **3**:27, 1975.
7. Gallagher, J. J., Sealy, W. C., Wallace, A. G., and Kasell, J.: Correlation between catheter electrophysiological studies and findings on mapping of ventricular excitation in the WPW syndrome. In Wellens, H. J. J., Lie, K. I., and Janse, M. J., editors: The conduction system of the heart, Philadelphia, 1976, Lea & Febiger.
8. Lev, M.: Anatomical basis for pre-excitation, Second International Symposium on Clinical Electrophysiology, Chicago, May 10-12, 1978.
9. Coumel, P., and Attuel, P.: Reciprocating

tachycardia in overt and latent pre-excitation, Eur. J. Cardiol. **1**:423, 1974.

10. Wellens, H. J. J.: Electrophysiology and mechanism of supraventricular tachycardia in WPW, Second International Symposium on Clinical Electrophysiology, Chicago, May 10-12, 1978.

11. Sung, P. J., Gelband, H., Castellanos, A., Aranda, J. M., and Myerburf, R. J.: Clinical and electrophysiologic observations in patients with concealed accessory atrioventricular bypass tracts, Am. J. Cardiol. **40**:839, 1977.

12. Wolff, L., Parkinson, J., and White, P. D.: Bundle-branch block with short P-R interval in healthy young people prone to paroxysmal tachycardia, Am. Heart. J. **5**:685, 1930.

13. Kent, A. F. S.: Researches on structure and function of mammalian heart, J. Physiol. **14**: 233, 1893.

14. Paladino, G.: Contribuzione all'anatomia, istologia e fisiologia del cuore, Mov. Med.-Chir. (Napoli) **8**:428, 1876.

15. Holzman, M., and Scherf, D.: Uber Elektrokardiogramme mit vorkurzten vorhol Kammer-Distanz und positiven P-Zacken, Z. Klin. Med. **121**:404, 1932.

16. Wolferth, C. C., and Wood, F. C.: The mechanism of production of short P-R intervals and prolonged QRS complexes in patients with presumably undamaged hearts. Hypothesis of an accessory pathway of auriculoventricular conduction (bundle of Kent), Am. Heart. J. **8**:297, 1933.

17. Wood, F. C., Wolferth, C. C., and Geckeler, G. D.: Histological demonstration of accessory muscular connections between auricle and ventricle in a case of short P-R interval and prolonged QRS complex, Am. Heart. J. **25**:454, 1943.

18. Ohnell, R. F.: Preexcitation, a cardiac abnormality, Acta Med. Scand. **152**(supp.):74, 1944.

19. Durrer, D., and Wellens, H. J. J.: The Wolff-Parkinson-White syndrome anno 1973, Eur. J. Cardiol. **1**:367, 1974.

20. Wellens, H. J. J.: Electrical stimulation of the heart in the study of tachycardias, Baltimore, 1971, University Park Press.

21. Zipes, D. P., Rothbaum, D. A., and DeJoseph, R. L.: Preexcitation syndrome, Cardiovasc. Clin. **6**:210, 1975.

22. Wellens, H. J. J., Farre, J., and Bar, F. W. H. M.: The WPW syndrome. In Mandel, W.: Management of difficult arrhythmias, J. B. Lippincott Co. (In press).

23. Gomes, J. A. C., and Haft, J. I.: Wolff-Parkinson-White syndrome type B with His depolarization occurring after the QRS: further evidence that WPW-QRS is a fusion beat, Chest **67**:445, 1975.

24. Wellens, H. J. J.: Electrophysiology of WPW syndrome. In Wellens, H. J. J., Lie, K. I., and Janse, M. J., editors: The conduction system of the heart, Philadelphia, 1976, Lea Febiger.

25. Rosenbaum, M. B., Hecht, H. H., Wilson F. H., et al.: The potential variations of the thorax and the esophagus in anomalous atrioventricular excitation (Wolff-Parkinson-White syndrome), Am. Heart J. **29**:281, 1945.

26. Durrer, D., and Roos, J. P.: Epicardial excitation of the ventricles in a patient with Wolff-Parkinson-White syndrome (type B) Circulation **35**:15, 1967.

27. Wallace, A. G., Sealy, W. C., Gallagher, J. J., Svenson, R. H., Strauss, H. C., and Kasseł J.: Surgical correction of anomalous left ventricular preexcitation: Wolff-Parkinson-White (type A): Circulation **49**:206, 1974.

28. Durrer, D., Schoo, L., Schuilenburg, R. M., and Wellens, H. J. J.: The role of premature beats in the initiation and termination of supraventricular tachycardia in the Wolff-Parkinson-White syndrome, Circulation **36**: 644, 1967.

29. Laham, J.: Le syndrome de Wolff-Parkinson-White, Paris, 1969, Librairie Maloine.

30. Campbell, R. W. F., Smith, R. A., Gallagher, J. J., Prichett, E. L. C., and Wallace, A. G.: Atrial fibrillation in the preexcitation syndrome, Am. J. Cardiol. **40**:514, 1977.

31. Sung, R. J., Gelband, H., Castellanos, A., Aranda, J. M., and Myerburf, R. J.: Clinical and electrophysiologic observations in patients with concealed accessory atrioventricular bypass tracts, Am. J. Cardiol. **40**:839, 1977.

32. Lown, B., Ganong, W. F., and Levine, S. A.: The syndrome of short P-R interval, normal QRS complex and paroxysmal rapid heart action, Circulation **5**:696, 1952.

33. Sherf, L.: The atrial conduction system: clinical implications, Am. J. Cardiol. **37**:814, 1976.

34. Caracta, A. R., Damato, A. N., Gallagher, J. J., et al.: Electrophysiological studies in the syndrome short P-R interval, normal QRS complex, Am. J. Cardiol. **31**:245, 1973.

35. Josephson, M. E., and Kastor, J. A.: Supra

ventricular tachycardia in Lown-Ganong-Levine syndrome: atrionodal versus intranodal reentry. Amer. J. Cardiol. **40:**521, 1977.

6. Mahaim, I., and Winston, R. M.: Recherches d'anatomie comparee et de pathologie experimentale sur les connexions hautes du faisceau de His-Tawara, Cardiologia **5:**189, 1941.

7. Mahaim, I.: Kent's fibers and the A-V paraspecific conduction through the upper connections of the bundle of His-Tawara, Am. Heart J. **33:**651, 1947.

8. Wellens, H. J. J., Lubbers, W. J., and Losekoot, T. G.: Preexcitation. In Roberts, N. K., and Gelband, H., editors: Cardiac arrhythmias in the neonate, infant, and child. New York, 1977, Appleton-Century-Crofts.

39. Coumel, P., Waynberger, M., and Fabiato, A.: Wolff-Parkinson-White syndrome. Problems in evaluation of multiple accessory pathway and surgical therapy, Circulation **45:**1216, 1972.

40. Josephson, M. E., Caracta, A. R., Lau, S. H., et al.: Alternating type A and type B Wolff-Parkinson-White syndrome, Am. Heart J. **87:** 363, 1974.

41. Spurrell, R. A. J., Krikler, D. M., and Sowton, E.: Problems concerning assessment of anatomical site of accessory pathway in Wolff-Parkinson-White syndrome, Br. Heart J. **37:** 127, 1978.

CHAPTER 14

Fusion complexes

In electrocardiography the term *fusion* is used to indicate that two vec tors from two different foci that have started to move at almost the sam time have met within the muscle mass of either the ventricle (ventricular fu sion) or the atrium (atrial fusion). Contrary to what is sometimes though the term *fusion beat* does not mean that a P wave has occurred during th QRS complex.

Electrophysiology

The terms *atrial fusion* or *ventricular fusion* imply that there are two vec tors or currents active simultaneously within the atria or ventricles. Thes two vectors simply cancel each other out, causing a complex of lower ampli tude. Fig. 14-1 shows that when the depolarization process is initiated fron two different sites within the atria or the ventricles, opposing cell masse become immediately negative, thus making it impossible for a large numbe of negative ions to oppose a large number of positive ions. Therefore th vector can never at any moment in the process be very big, since it is th

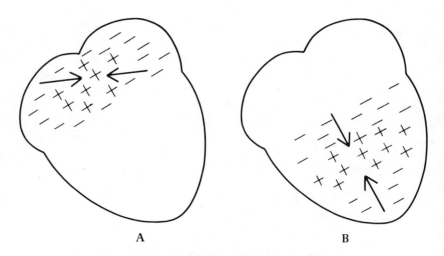

Fig. 14-1. A, Atrial fusion. **B,** Ventricular fusion.

number of negative cells opposing positive cells that determines the strength of the vector.

Atrial fusion beats occur most frequently when an ectopic atrial focus and the sinus node discharge simultaneously or almost simultaneously (Fig. 14-1, *A*). Ventricular fusion beats most often occur when an ectopic ventricular focus discharges at the same or almost the same time that normal conduction begins at the AV junction (Fig. 14-1, *B*).

ECG changes

1. *Complexes of low amplitude:* Complexes of low amplitude are caused by two smaller vectors canceling each other out.
2. *Complexes of shorter duration:* Complexes of shorter duration are seen both in P fusion and in QRS fusion beats. Two electrical forces cause the depolarization process to be completed more quickly.

Ventricular fusion

In the tracing shown in Fig. 14-2 an end-diastolic PVC is not early enough to completely capture the ventricle. The ectopic vector begins to activate the ventricle at almost the same time that the normal vector has begun its course down the IV septum. The electrical forces thus cancel each other out, and a complex of lesser amplitude is produced. The duration of the depolarization process has been shortened from 0.12 to 0.05 sec. Notice also that the aberrant ventricular activity has caused an aberrant T wave.

Ventricular fusion beats are often seen at the beginning and end of the accelerated idioventricular rhythm. Because the idioventricular rhythm is of-

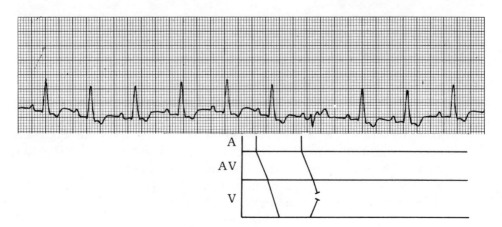

Fig. 14-2. Ventricular fusion.

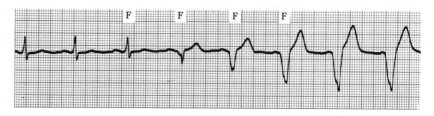

Fig. 14-3. Accelerated idioventricular rhythm. Note the changing shape of the fusion beats, *F*, as the ventricular ectopic focus dominates more completely with each beat.

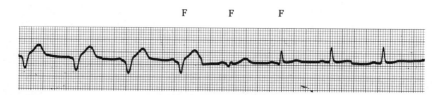

Fig. 14-4. An accelerated idioventricular rhythm. Note the three fusion beats, *F*, as the sinus-conducted impulse captures more and more of the ventricles until finally the ventricular ectopic focus is closed out altogether.

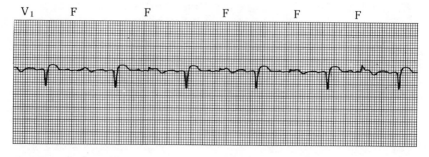

Fig. 14-5. Bigeminal end-diastolic PVCs that are all fusion beats, *F*. (From Conover, M. H.: Cardiac arrhythmias: exercises in pattern interpretation, ed. 2, St. Louis, 1978, The C. V. Mosby Co.)

ten approximately the same rate as that of the sinus node, if the sinus node slows down just a little bit, the ventricular ectopic focus discharges at the same time, and the two forces collide within the ventricle. Fig. 14-3 illustrates such a rhythm. The first two beats are probably totally sinus conducted. But notice the subtle difference in shape of the third beat, a difference that you would not even notice were it not for what followed. The next three beats are also fusion beats. Note how the ectopic forces dominate more and more in each successive beat as the sinus-conducted impulse loses control of the ventricles.

Fig. 14-4 illustrates the end of an accelerated idioventricular rhythm from another patient.

There probably isn't another tracing as confusing to look at as is the bigeminal end-diastolic PVC, since these beats are usually fusion beats. Such a tracing is seen in Fig. 14-5. Some complexes are so isoelectric that only the T wave can be seen. If you walk out the P waves, you will find them to be right on time.

Summary

Fusion beats can occur within the atria or ventricles and are the result of two opposing currents within the same chamber. These two different currents originate from two different places in the heart; usually one is normal and the other ectopic. This collision of forces results in an ECG complex that is neither normal nor looks like the ectopic beat but is something in between, often narrower and of lesser amplitude than either the normal or the ectopic.

CHAPTER 15

Hypertrophies

Left ventricular hypertrophy

When the left ventricle hypertrophies, the disproportion in size between the left and right ventricles is further increased and causes greater amplitude in the ECG deflections, but a normal sequence of depolarization is retained.

ECG changes

1. *QRS amplitude:* The increase in the amplitude of the main ventricular vector is best reflected in the precordial leads. In leads facing the hypertrophied ventricle (V_6), a tall R wave (17 mm or more) is usually present. In leads facing the negative side of the activation (V_1), a deep S wave is seen. The R wave in V_5 or V_6, plus the S wave in V_1 or V_2, often are in excess of 40 mm.

2. *QRS duration:* The QRS interval lasts as long as the depolarization wave spreads through the ventricles (0.09 sec or more). Prolongation of the QRS therefore represents delayed conduction of the impulse through the ventricles. In the presence of left ventricular hypertrophy, delay is caused by the presence of more ventricular muscle tissue. A longer time is necessary for the current to completely depolarize the thickened muscle.

3. *Ventricular activation time (VAT):* In the thickened left ventricle a longer time is required for the current to reach the epicardium. Therefore in leads facing the left ventricle (V_6), the peak of the R wave is delayed (0.05 sec or more), as shown in Fig. 15-1.

4. *T waves:* These may be of polarity opposite to that of the main QRS deflection. The repolarization process is changed because of delayed conduction through the ventricles.

5. *S-T segment displacement:* This displacement is in a direction opposite to that of the main QRS deflection.

6. *Left atrial involvement:* This may be associated with left ventricular hypertrophy and would be reflected in V_1 as a P wave with a terminal negative deflection of 1 mm or more and a duration of 0.04 sec or more (Fig. 15-2).

7. *Left axis deviation:* A deviation of -30 degrees or more may be present.

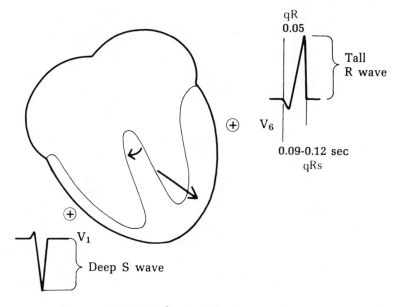

Fig. 15-1. Left ventricular hypertrophy.

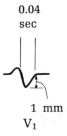

Fig. 15-2. Abnormal P wave in association with left ventricular hypertrophy.

Left ventricular strain

The term *strain* is used to describe the ST-T changes that sometimes are seen with left ventricular hypertrophy. Its exact etiology is unknown; however, it has been known to be associated with long-standing left ventricular hypertrophy. It will intensify when myocardial dilatation and failure occur. The strain pattern is composed of the following: depressed, convex ST segment and inverted T waves in leads V_5, V_6, I, and aVL.

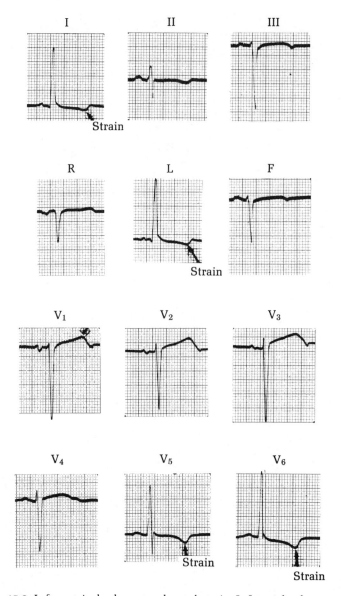

Fig. 15-3. Left ventricular hypertrophy and strain. Left atrial enlargement.

Fig. 15-3 reflects left ventricular hypertrophy and strain. The following diagnostic features can be noted in this ECG:

1. *QRS amplitude:* The R wave in V_1 plus the S wave in V_6 are greater than 40 mm.
2. *QRS duration:* 0.10 sec.
3. *Ventricular activation time in V_6:* 0.05 sec.

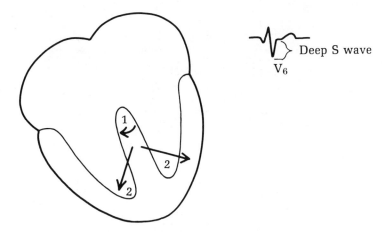

Fig. 15-4. Right ventricular hypertrophy.

4. Typical ST and T waves changes.
5. *Left atrial involvement:* Note the P wave in V_1. Its terminal deflection is negative with a duration of more than 0.04 sec and an amplitude of 1 mm.
6. *Left axis deviation.*
7. *Strain.* The left ventricular strain pattern is noted in leads V_5, V_6, I and aV_1.

Right ventricular hypertrophy

Normally the electrical forces of the thick left ventricle dominate the ECG. When the right ventricle hypertrophies, this vectorial supremacy shifts. Therefore leads facing the right ventricle (V_1 and V_2) resemble left ventricular leads. Conversely, the left ventricular leads (V_5 and V_6) reflect ECG patterns that are ordinarily seen in right ventricular leads (Fig. 15-4).

ECG changes

1. *Precordial leads:* The configuration of the precordial leads is reversed so that those facing the right ventricle have tall R waves. Leads facing the left ventricle have small r and deep S waves that reflect the dominance of the hypertrophied right ventricle.
2. *QRS duration:* The interval does not increase in duration. Even though the right ventricular wall is hypertrophied, it rarely exceeds the normal thickness of the left ventricular wall. Therefore the depolarization process does not take longer. Both ventricles will have completed the depolarization process at approximately the same time.
3. *T wave:* The T wave is of opposite polarity to the main QRS deflection. This usually occurs when there is a change in the depolarization forces.

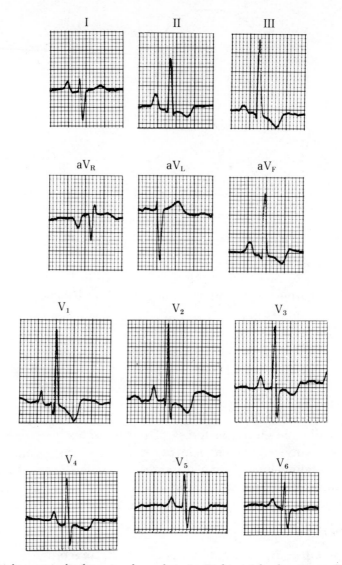

Fig. 15-5. Right ventricular hypertrophy and strain. Right atrial enlargement. (From Conover, M.: Cardiac arrhythmias: exercises in pattern interpretation, ed. 2, St. Louis, 1978, The C. V. Mosby Co.)

4. *Right atrial involvement:* This may be associated with right ventricular hypertrophy and would be reflected as tall, peaked P waves in leads II and III.

5. *Right axis deviation.*

6. *Strain:* A strain pattern is seen in leads facing the right ventricle (a depressed, convex ST segment and inverted T wave).

Fig. 15-5 reflects right ventricular hypertrophy and strain. Note the following diagnostic features in the ECG:

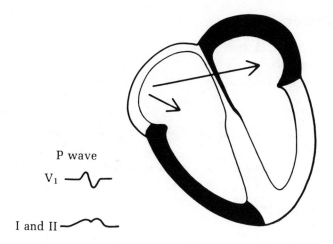

Fig. 15-6. Left atrial hypertrophy.

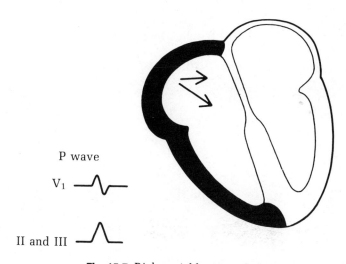

Fig. 15-7. Right atrial hypertrophy.

a. *Precordial leads:* Note the tall R waves in V_1 and V_2 and the deep S wave in V_6.
b. *QRS duration:* The QRS duration is 0.08 sec (normal).
c. *T waves.* The T waves are of opposite polarity to the main QRS.
d. *Right atrial involvement:* This is reflected by tall peaked P waves in lead II.
e. *Right axis deviation.*
f. *Strain:* A strain pattern is seen in V_1 to V_4.

Left atrial hypertrophy

Left atrial hypertrophy is often accompanied by right ventricular hypertrophy, particularly when it occurs secondary to mitral stenosis, one of the more common causes of left atrial enlargement (Figs. 15-3 and 15-6).

ECG changes

1. *Leads I and II:* "P mitrale" (broad notched P wave—more than 0.11 sec in duration).
2. *Lead V_1:* Diphasic P wave with a broad, terminal, negative deflection.

Right atrial hypertrophy

Right atrial hypertrophy is often caused by chronic pulmonary disease and is frequently accompanied by a hypertrophied right ventricle (Figs 15-5 and 15-7).

ECG changes

1. *Leads II and III:* "P pulmonale" (tall, peaked P wave more than 2.5 mm in height).
2. *Lead V_1:* Upright P wave, tall and peaked.

CHAPTER 16

Pacemakers

History

In 1952 Zoll[1] was the first to use external electrical stimuli to resuscitate a heart in ventricular standstill.

In 1958 Furman,[2] then a hospital resident, and Robinson published an article on the feasibility of long-term transvenous pacing. Five years later Lagergren and Johansson[3] (in Sweden) described permanent transvenous pacing of the heart.

The first permanent pacemakers were implanted in 1959 by Senning[4] in Europe and Hunter[5] in the United States.

Prior to the discovery and use of pacemakers, complete heart block was associated with a mortality rate of 50% after one year and 90% after five years.[6] Now, for those patients who are under 65 years of age at implantation, 50% will survive for more than 10 years, and 25% to 30% of all patients, irrespective of age, will also survive that long. Not only does the pacemaker alleviate the symptoms of bradycardia, but also it has been successfully used to terminate atrial and ventricular tachyarrhythmias by rapid intra-cardiac stimuli.[7-9] Medical technology continues to improve circuitry, energy source, performance, and programability of pacemakers.

Types of pacemakers

Before 1964 all pacemakers discharged at a fixed rate, making nomenclature simple. After that time, not only was the demand pacemaker introduced but also the paced and sensed chambers, and there were many brand names for the same pacemaker. In an attempt to sort out the resulting confused nomenclature, three noted authorities published a suggested three-letter identification code for implantable cardiac pacemakers.[10]

The first letter of this code identifies the paced chamber: V = ventricle, A = atrium, and D = double (atrium and ventricle).

The second letter identifies the sensed chamber: A or V.

The third letter identifies the mode of response: I = inhibited and T = triggered.

The letter O indicates that the specific comment is not applicable. For

Table 2. Suggested nomenclature code for implantable cardiac pacemakers*

Chamber paced	Chamber sensed	Mode of response	Generic description	Previously used designation
V	O	O	Ventricular pacing; no sensing function	Asynchronous; fixed rate; set rate
A	O	O	Atrial pacing; no sensing function	Atrial fixed rate; atrial asynchronous
D	O	O	Atrioventricular pacing; no sensing function	AV sequential; fixed rate; asynchronous
V	V	I	Ventricular pacing and sensing; inhibited mode	Ventricular inhibited; R inhibited; R blocking; R suppressed; noncompetitive inhibited; demand; standby
V	V	T	Ventricular pacing and sensing; triggered mode	Ventricular triggered; R triggered; R wave stimulated; noncompetitive triggered; following; R synchronous; demand; standby
A	A	I	Atrial pacing and sensing; inhibited mode	Atrial inhibited; P inhibited; P blocking; P suppressed
A	A	T	Atrial pacing and sensing; triggered mode	Atrial triggered; P triggered; P stimulated; P synchronous
V	A	T	Ventricular pacing, atrial sensing; triggered mode	Atrial synchronous; atrial synchronous, AV synchronous
D	V	I	Atrioventricular pacing, ventricular sensing; inhibited mode	Bifocal sequential demand; AV sequential

*From Parsonnet, V., Furman, S., and Smyth, N. P. D.: Implantable cardiac pacemakers: status report and resource guideline, Am. J. Cardiol. **34:**489, 1974.
Key: V = ventricle, A = atrium, D = double (atrium and ventricle), I = inhibited, T = triggered, O = specific comment not applicable.

example, *VOO* would indicate ventricular pacing with no sensing function (fixed-rate; asynchronous).

Table 2 explains this suggested nomenclature code and gives a generic description of the different types of pacemakers, as well as listing previously used descriptions.

Fixed-rate pacemakers (AOO, VOO, and DOO) maintain a constant rate, which may compete with natural cardiac activity. The ECG from such a pacemaker is seen in Fig. 16-1. Such competition becomes a hazard when the threshold for ventricular fibrillation is low, as it is immediately after myocardial infarction.

The QRS-inhibited pacemaker (VVI) is a demand pacemaker with the

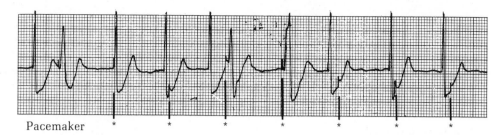

Fig. 16-1. Fixed-rate pacemaker in competition with the patient's own rhythm.

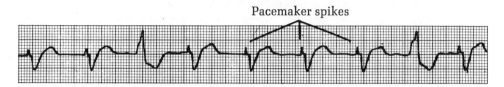

Fig. 16-2. QRS-inhibited pacemaker (VVI).

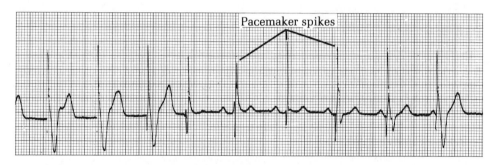

Fig. 16-3. QRS-triggered pacemaker (VVI).

inhibited mode of response; that is, such a pacemaker does not fire when sensing an R wave. The ECG from the QRS-inhibited pacemaker is seen in Fig. 16-2.

The QRS-triggered pacemaker (VVT) is a demand pacemaker with the triggered mode of response; that is, such a pacemaker senses the R wave and fires in the absolute refractory period. Thus as long as there is an adequate natural cardiac rhythm, there is a pacemaker spike but no cardiac response. If the natural cardiac rate falls below the preset rate of the pacemaker, the artificial discharge then captures the myocardium. The ECG from a QRS-triggered pacemaker is seen in Fig. 16-3.

Atrial synchronized pacing (VAT) requires an atrial electrode, which senses normal atrial depolarization. A ventricular electrode is then triggered to pace the ventricle after an appropriate delay to allow for atrial transport.

Atrioventricular sequential pacing (DVI) requires the pacing of both the atrium and the ventricle by two separate electrodes acting in sequence. This pacemaker is inhibited by ventricular activity.

Pacing system

The pacing electrode, consisting of a negative and a positive pole, is attached by wire to the pulse generator. When the pulse generator discharges, an electrical current flows between these two poles. The generator is powered by an energy source, usually lithium, mercury-zinc, or nuclear.

The electrode may be unipolar or bipolar. These terms refer to the number of electrodes in contact with the myocardium. In a unipolar system the intracardiac electrode is the positive one (cathode), while the negative electrode (anode) is outside the heart, buried in subcutaneous tissue.

In a bipolar system, both electrodes lie against the myocardium. Two insulated conductors link the two electrodes to the pulse generator.

Pacemaker spikes

The ECG records the firing of the pacemaker as a spike (artifact), which is either sharp and narrow or broader and biphasic. The sharp, narrow spike

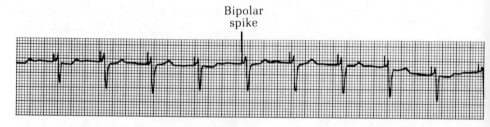

Fig. 16-4. Bipolar pacemaker spike.

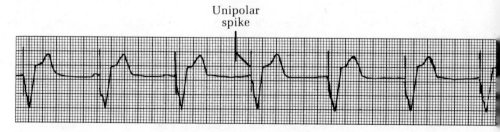

Fig. 16-5. Unipolar pacemaker spike.

may be either positive or negative, depending on the recording lead. The spike for a bipolar pacemaker is small (Fig. 16-4). The spike from a unipolar pacemaker is large (Fig. 16-5).

Ventricular complexes produced by the pacemaker spike

If the tip of the pacemaker catheter lies in the apex of the right ventricle, a left bundle branch pattern results (Fig. 16-6).

If the pacemaker electrode is implanted in the left ventricle, a right bundle branch pattern results (Fig. 16-7).

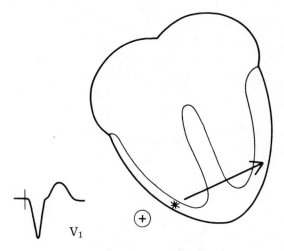

Fig. 16-6. Ventricular complex with the pacemaker electrode in the right ventricle.

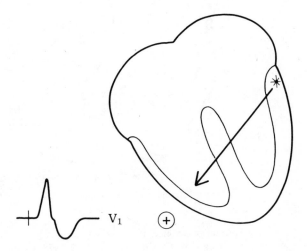

Fig. 16-7. Ventricular complex with the pacemaker electrode in the left ventricle.

Pacemaker fusion beats

When the pacemaker fires at the same time that a supraventricular impulse enters the ventricles, the two forces simultaneously depolarize the ventricles, resulting in a fusion beat. Such a complex is seen in Fig. 16-8.

F

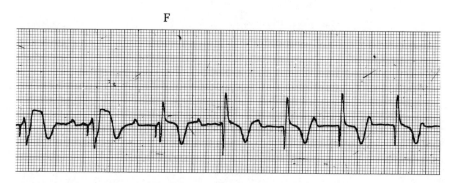

Fig. 16-8. Pacemaker fusion beat, *F*.

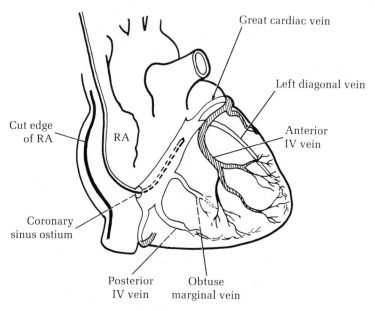

Fig. 16-9. Pacemaker catheter positioned in the coronary sinus. (From Greenberg, P., Castellanet, M., Messenger, J., and Ellestad, M. H.: Circulation **57**:98, 1978. By permission of the American Heart Association, Inc.)

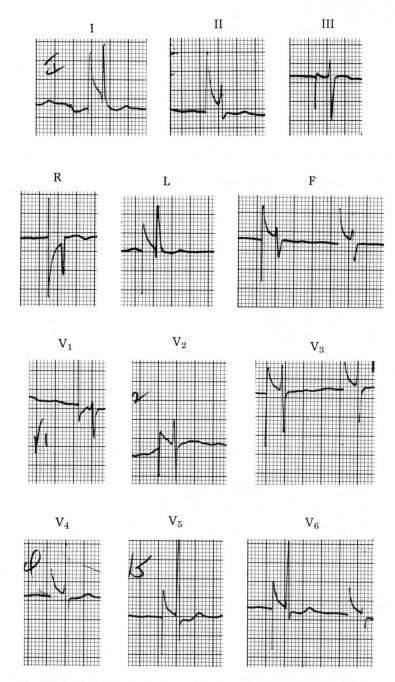

Fig. 16-10. Twelfth-lead ECG from a patient with a pacemaker in the coronary sinus. (Courtesy Dr. S. Serge Barold.)

Rate hysteresis

When a demand pacemaker is being used, the escape interval following a sensed beat is usually the same as the interval between impulses during continuous pacing. If the escape interval is significantly longer than that between two paced beats, the term *rate hysteresis* is used. This is a feature built in by the manufacturer in the hope that such a delay might take advantage of the atrial transport mechanism.

Pacemaker refractory period

All demand pacemakers have a built-in, artificial refractory period. During this time (usually 50 to 400 msec), following either a pacemaker discharge or a natural cardiac beat, the sensing circuit is insensitive to another signal. For atrial and coronary sinus pacing, the longer refractory period is required to avoid sensing the QRS complex.

Indications for a ventricular pacemaker

Symptomatic bradycardia remains the main indication for pacemaker insertion, with 85% of all pacemakers being used for this purpose. Whether or not the pacemaker is temporary or permanent will depend upon the cause of the bradycardia.

Pacemakers are also being successfully used in the treatment of sick sinus syndrome and atrial and ventricular tachyarrhythmias.[8,9,14]

Indications for atrial synchronous (VAT) pacing

The VAT pacemaker is commonly used when an atrial pacemaker is contraindicated because of the presence of complete heart block and when a ventricular pacemaker is contraindicated because the patient requires the hemodynamic benefit of atrial contraction preceding ventricular contraction.

Indications for atrial pacing (AAI, AAT)

An atrial pacemaker may be used whenever AV conduction is intact, and pacing is indicated. The difficulty lies in maintaining the electrode in contact with the atrial tissue. This problem may be overcome with the development of reliable lead fixation.

Atrial pacing is especially indicated for symptomatic bradycardia and the tachycardia-bradycardia syndrome (sick sinus syndrome) with intact AV conduction, with or without congestive failure and low cardiac output.

Rapid atrial pacing has also been reported to successfully terminate intractable supraventricular[8,9] and ventricular tachyarrhythmias.

Advantages of atrial pacing

Atrial pacing is hemodynamically superior to ventricular pacing in that the atrial contribution to ventricular filling is maintained,[14] and thus there is a greater improvement in ventricular performance.[15,16]

Atrial pacing from the coronary sinus

Pervenous atrial pacing from the coronary sinus is the most popular type of atrial pacing because such a site confines the pacemaker electrode so that it remains in contact with the atrial tissue. Fig. 16-9 illustrates a pacemaker catheter positioned in the coronary sinus. The ECG from such a patient is shown in Fig. 16-10.

Problems of pervenous atrial pacing and their solutions[17]

1. Threshold rise is manifested by loss of capture and corrected by reprograming the pacemaker from medium to high current output.
2. Migration of the catheter is manifested by loss of capture and corrected by repositioning the lead.
3. Failure of the pacer electrode to sense or capture following the onset of atrial fibrillation is corrected by electrical or drug cardioversion of the atrial fibrillation.
4. Dislodgment of the lead from the coronary sinus is manifested by loss of capture and corrected by reinsertion of the pacer.

How to test the functions of the demand pacemaker[11,12]

The two functions of the demand pacemaker, pacing and sensing, should be tested individually. Initially the pacing electrode should be positioned in the ventricle so that the least possible stimulus is required to pace the heart (low threshold). However, sometimes a position that is optimal for pacing is not good for sensing, and a compromise must be reached by repositioning the catheter.

HOW TO EVALUATE THE PACING FUNCTION[11]

When a demand pacemaker is suppressed by a spontaneous rhythm, one cannot be certain that the pacemaker will pace when required. Application of a magnet is the method of choice for testing the pacing function. Most

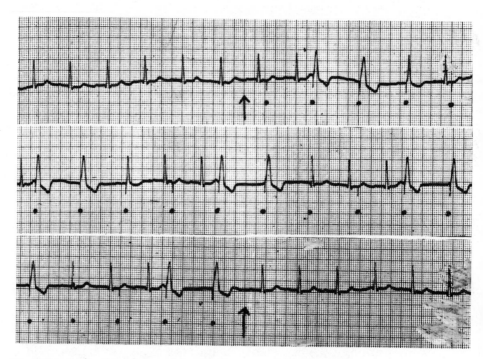

Fig. 16-11. Application of a special magnet on an implanted 5842 Medtronic demand pacemaker. At the beginning of the tracing the spontaneous rhythm is suppressed by the pacemaker. At the first arrow (magnet application) the pacemaker emits stimuli at a fixed rate (black dots). All stimuli outside the refractory period of the heart (QRS to apex of T wave) capture the ventricles. The magnet was removed at the second arrow (From Barold, S. S.: Heart Lung **2**[2]: 238, 1973.)

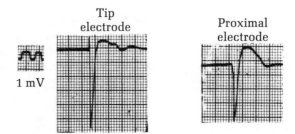

Fig. 16-12. Unipolar ventricular electrogram from the tip and proximal electrodes demonstrates the typical morphology seen at the right ventricular apex. Note the absence of recordable P wave voltage. The S-T segment elevation (current of injury) indicates good endocardial contact. The voltage of the unipolar electrograms from the tip electrode exceeds 12 mV and the one from the proximal electrode measures about 8 mV. (From Barold, S. S.: Heart Lung **2**[2]:238, 1973.)

demand pacemakers have a built-in switch by which they can be converted to a fixed-rate mode with the application of a special testing magnet. Fig. 16-11 illustrates the results of such a maneuver.

Carotid sinus pressure suppresses the spontaneous rhythm and is sometimes used to demonstrate the pacing capability of an implanted generator. However, this method carries with it all the risks of the maneuver itself, plus the fact that one has suppressed the spontaneous rhythm without knowing if the pacemaker can perform or not.

HOW TO EVALUATE THE SENSING FUNCTION[11-13]

Most demand pacemakers sense voltages as low as 2 to 3 mV as long as the signal resembles a QRS complex. However, the lowest effective intracardiac voltage should not be less than 5 mV.[11,12] This is measured by means of a *ventricular electrogram*, easily recorded on a standard ECG. One must, however, be absolutely certain that the equipment being used is well grounded in order to avoid accidental electrocution of the patient. See p. 253 concerning how to avoid accidental electrocution and p. 190 for tips on how to minimize the danger to the patient.

With the unipolar system a ventricular electrogram is recorded by connecting the V lead to the tip electrode (cathode) and then to the proximal electrode (anode). An example of the recording obtained is displayed in Fig. 16-12. The voltage available for sensing is the difference in potential between the two electrodes. However, in the unipolar system, since the voltage from the anodal electrode in the subcutaneous tissue contributes little to the total signal, the cathode (tip) from the intracardiac site closely reflects the signal available for sensing. In the example shown in Fig. 16-12, this signal exceeds 12 mV.

With the bipolar system a ventricular electrogram is recorded by connecting the ECG cables from lead I (right and left arms) to the tip and proximal electrodes of the pacing catheter. An example of the recording obtained is displayed in Fig. 16-13.

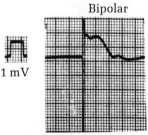

Bipolar

1 mV

Fig. 16-13. Ventricular electrogram from a bipolar pacing catheter with electrodes 2 cm apart. The largest defective bipolar voltage from bottom to top measures 8 mV. (From Barold, S. S.: Heart Lung **2**[2]:238, 1973.)

OTHER USES OF THE VENTRICULAR ELECTROGRAM[15-17]

1. To determine the location of the catheter (A well-wedged catheter in the right ventricular apex has an rS pattern of from 5 to 15 mV with small or absent P waves whereas a catheter in the coronary sinus has peaked high-voltage P waves on the ventricular electrogram.)
2. To determine good endocardial contact and a low threshold for pacing as manifest by S-T segment elevation (current of injury)

HOW TO EVALUATE THE DEMAND MODE AND INHERENT HEART RHYTHM DURING APPARENT FIXED-RATE PACING[11]

Under the circumstances just described, one could apply chest wall stimulation. The signals from a standard external pulse generator are too weak to affect the heart but may completely suppress the implanted pacemaker, thus testing its demand property while creating an opportunity to visualize the patient's inherent rhythm for diagnostic changes.

How to protect the patient from accidental electrocution during temporary pacing

Because the pacing catheter bridges the protective resistance of the skin and offers a direct line to the myocardium, extreme caution is necessary when caring for a patient with temporary pacing. This is most especially true when performing the ventricular electrogram, in which case an electrically powered piece of equipment (ECG machine) is connected directly to the pacing catheter. Currents below 1 mA and even as low as 10 μA may cause ventricular fibrillation when applied directly to the myocardium through the pacing catheter. Currents as low as this are imperceptible if applied to the skin. Therefore if a danger to the patient does exist, *the operating personnel are unable to detect it.* Periodic inspection of equipment is therefore absolutely necessary. This inspection should be of such a quality as to ensure proper grounding and minimal leakage currents. Please refer to Chapter 19 for a more complete discussion on this subject.

Additionally, the following should be observed[12]:

1. The power line must have a three-wire cord terminating in a three-prong, heavy-duty plug for proper grounding between the chassis and the alternating current (AC) ground.
2. The pacemaker should be battery operated.
3. The ECG amplifiers should have isolated inputs.
4. No other electrically operated equipment should be attached to the patient.
5. The patient should be kept isolated from ground if possible.
6. Never touch a terminal with your bare hands.

7. Never allow the terminal to be in contact with liquids or metal objects.
8. Insulate a free terminal carefully with tape and secure it firmly.
9. Isolate the entire pacemaker and terminals inside a rubber surgical glove.

Methods of insertion

The pacemaker electrode can be placed in contact with the myocardium by the transvenous, epicardial, or transthoracic method.

TRANSVENOUS METHOD

A transvenous pacemaker may be temporary or permanent. An electrode catheter is placed in the apex of the right ventricle in close contact with the endocardial surface. The catheter is inserted under fluoroscopic control. A cutdown or percutaneous technique may be used. The pacing catheter that is threaded into the right ventricle may be introduced by way of the jugular, basilic, femoral, subclavian, or cephalic vein (Fig. 16-14). The temporary transvenous pacemaker is attached to an external battery unit, and the control battery of the permanent transvenous pacemaker is inserted surgically into the subcutaneous tissue of the chest.

Fig. 16-15 illustrates the commonly used cephalic vein insertion and pulse generator placement.

Most transvenous pacemakers are placed within the right ventricular cavity. However, the pacemaker catheter may be placed in the atrium if there is no pathological process in the AV node. The electrical events of the ventricles would then occur normally, synchronized with the atrial contraction. Cardiac output would be improved by this method, but the catheter position is somewhat less reliable.

EPICARDIAL METHOD

A thoracotomy is necessary for this procedure, in which electrodes are sutured to the epicardium. The pulse generator is buried in a subcutaneous pocket. The pacing mode may be either synchronous or asynchronous.

The electrode may be sutured to or screwed into the myocardium by a number of routes. These surgical approaches are illustrated in Fig. 16-16. The left subcostal approach is preferred over an upper abdominal midline incision and a transxiphisternal incision for the sutureless electrode (corkscrew configuration) because with this exposure the electrode can be implanted into the left ventricle, whereas in the other approaches only the right ventricle is available. The left ventricle is superior to the right for pacing because it is thicker and therefore more suitable for the corkscrew implant and because the electrogram from the left ventricle is stronger and

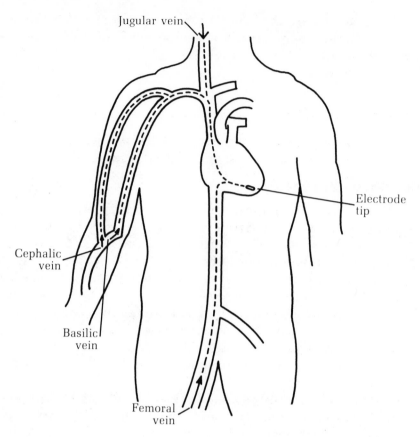

Fig. 16-14. Routes commonly used to introduce a transvenous pacemaker into the right ventricle.

more easily sensed by the electrode. The sutureless electrode may also be implanted with left anterolateral thoracotomy (Fig. 16-16).

A major indication for the epicardial method is the occasional inability of the transvenous electrode to remain seated (in contact with the endocardium). This is especially true when the right ventricle is dilated and smooth walled.

TRANSTHORACIC METHOD

A large needle is used to insert the electrodes directly into the ventricle through the chest wall. This is an emergency procedure and can be lifesaving. Possible complications include pneumothorax, damage to a coronary artery, tamponade, unstable pacing, or electrode displacement. The last two are particular dangers if closed-chest massage is in progress.

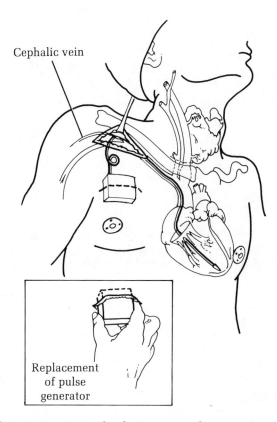

Fig. 16-15. Cephalic vein insertion and pulse generator placement. (From Furman, S.: Heart Lung **7**[5]:813, 1978.)

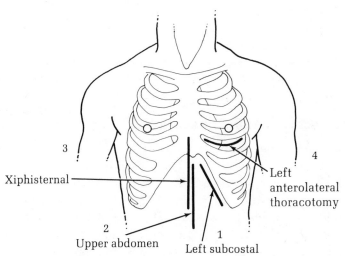

Fig. 16-16. Surgical approaches for the epicardial pacemaker. (From Furman, S.: Heart Lung **7**[5]:822, 1978.)

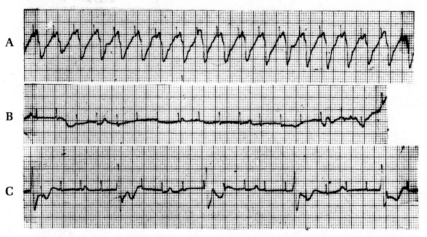

Fig. 16-17. Medtronic "runaway" fixed-rate pacemaker (1969). The pacemaker rate of about 170 beats/min results in artificial ventricular tachycardia. This was initially mistaken for true ventricular tachycardia for which lidocaine was administered. This led to Strip B where the pacemaker stimuli became ineffectual (presumably because lidocaine altered the threshold for pacing) and all underlying ventricular activity was eliminated. Strip C was recorded shortly afterward showing a slow idioventricular rhythm with ineffectual pacemaker spikes (From Barold, S. S.: Heart Lung **2**[2]:238, 1973.)

Pacemaker failure

Battery exhaustion is responsible for 80% to 90% of pacemaker failure. Following are the signs of battery failure:
1. Loss of capture
2. Poor intrinsic rhythm
3. Loss of demand function
4. Decrease in rate by 2 or 3 beats/min or more

The integrity of the pacemaker should be evaluated according to the separate functions of pacing and sensing.

ABNORMALITIES RELATED TO PACING[12]

Abnormalities related to pacing are (1) total failure to capture, (2) no pacemaker spikes on the ECG, and (3) abnormal firing (erratic or irregular).

Failure to capture is usually related to displacement or malplacement of the electrode, which may not be detected radiologically. It must be repositioned. If the electrode has perforated, it may first be noticed because of intercostal or diaphragmatic stimulation, pacemaker sound, pericardial rub, and/or a change from LBBB to RBBB pattern.

Lack of pacemaker spikes on the ECG may be due to total failure of the battery or components or to interruption of the electrical circuit (usually secondary to a broken electrode with intact insulation).

Abnormal firing may be due to component failure. Although decrease in stimulation rate is the usual result of battery depletion, *runaway pacemaker* is a rare but serious complication. Such an event requires immediate disconnection of the pacemaker. Fig. 16-17 illustrates a runaway pacemaker with a rate of about 170 beats/min. Rates as high as 400 beats/min may occur. Even if a pacemaker rate increases by only 10 to 15 beats/min, consider this an emergency, since very rapid rates could occur suddenly.[11]

ABNORMALITIES RELATED TO SENSING[11,12]

Undersensing

Loss of the specialized demand function is more common in bipolar systems than in unipolar ones because of the less reliable signals provided by the bipolar electrogram.

When a pacemaker fails to sense a previously normal QRS complex, it is usually due to catheter displacement, ischemia or extension of a myocardial infarction, development of intraventricular conduction delay (i.e., BBB) or alteration of the ventricular electrogram because of electrolyte imbalance or antiarrhythmic agents.

Oversensing

The pacing function of a demand pacemaker may be suppressed by signals from within or outside of the body. Signals from within the body include P and T wave voltage and afterpotentials from the pacemaker pulse.

P wave sensing indicates catheter displacement. T wave sensing usually occurs only with paced beats. This unwanted signal can usually be reduced by simply reducing the sensitivity control setting of an external demand pacemaker. If this is not possible, then one could either convert the system to unipolar or reverse the polarity of the electrodes. Do not increase the pacing rate as a compensatory measure, since oversensing may be intermittent and excessively rapid rates may result.

Afterpotentials from the pacemaker pulse (false signals) are not detected on the ECG but will result in chaotic patterns of pacing and sensing. A loose connection between the electrode and the pacemaker is the most common cause of false signals. Other causes are saline, sweat, or urine near the poles of the external pacemaker, each of which may cause a short circuit.

References

1. Zoll, P. M.: Resuscitation of the heart in ventricular standstill by external electrical stimulation, N. Engl. J. Med. **247**:768, 1952.
2. Furman, S., and Robinson, G.: Use of intracardiac pacemaker in correction of total heart block, Surg. Forum **9**:245, 1958.
3. Lagergren, H., and Johansson, L.: Intracardiac stimulation for complete heart block, Acta Chir. Scand. **125**:562, 1963.
4. Senning, A.: Discussion of Stephenson, S. E., Jr., Edwards, W. H., Jolly, P. C., and Scott, H. W., Jr.: Physiologic p-wave cardiac stimu-

lator, J. Thorac. Cardiovasc. Surg. **38:**369, 1959.

5. Hunter, S. W., Roth, N. A., Bernardez, D., et al.: A bipolar myocardial electrode for complete heart block, J. Lancet. **79:**506, 1959.

6. Parsonnet, V.: Permanent pacing of the heart: 1952 to 1976, Am. J. Cardiol. **39:**250, 1977.

7. Wyndham, C. R., Wu, D., Denes, P., Sugarman, D., Levitsky, H. S., and Rosen, K. M.: Self-initiated conversion of paroxysmal atrial flutter utilizing a radio-frequency pacemaker, Am. J. Cardiol. **41:**1119, 1978.

8. Das, G., Anand, K. M., et al.: Atrial pacing for cardioversion of atrial flutter in digitalized patients, Am. J. Cardiol. **41:**308, 1978.

9. Fisher, J. D., Mehra, R., and Furman, S.: Termination of ventricular tachycardia with bursts of rapid ventricular pacing, Am. J. Cardiol. **41:**94, 1978.

10. Parsonnet, V., Furman, S., and Smyth, N. P. D.: Implantable cardiac pacemakers: status report and resource guideline, Am. J. Cardiol. **34:**487, 1974.

11. Barold, S. S.: Modern concepts of cardiac pacing, Heart Lung **2:**238, 1973.

12. Barold, S. S.: Clinical problems with temporary ventricular pacing. In Furman, S., and Escher, D., editors: Modern cardiac pacing, a clinical overview, Bowie, Md, 1975, The Charles Press, Publishers.

13. Barold, S. S., and Gaidula, J. J.: Evaluation of normal and abnormal sensing functions of demand pacemakers, Am. J. Cardiol. **28:**201, 1971.

14. Barold, S. S.: Therapeutic uses of cardiac pacing and tachyarrhythmias in His bundle electrocardiography and clinical electrophysiology, In Narula, Q., editor: Philadelphia, 1975, F. A. Davis Co.

15. Martin, R. H., and Cobb, L. A.: Observations on the effect of atrial systole in man, J. Lab. Clin. Med. **68:**224, 1966.

16. Benchimol, A., Ellis, E. G., and Dimond, E. G.: Hemodynamic consequences of atrial with ventricular pacing in patients with normal and abnormal hearts, Am. J. Med. **39:**911, 1965.

17. Moss, A. J., and Rivers, R. J.: Atrial pacing from the coronary vein: ten year experience in 50 patients with implanted pervenous pacemakers, Circulation **57:**103, 1978.

CHAPTER 17

Myocardial infarction

The results of an occlusion of a coronary artery depend on the state of the collateral circulation and the location of the occlusion. Cellular changes begin immediately. Unless blood flow is reestablished to the ischemic tissue, more and more cells will succumb to the effects of anoxia. Approximately 20 minutes after the occlusion the first necrotic cells appear. Until this point, recovery would have been rapid with a reestablished blood flow, but necrosis is irreversible.

These irreversibly injured necrotic cells lie toward the center of the infarct. Surrounding this center is an area of tissue that is nonfunctional (injured). Ischemic, though functioning, tissue is closest to the normally perfused areas at the periphery.

These histological changes in the myocardium are reflected in the ECG patterns shown in Fig. 17-1. Inverted T waves that are typically symmetrical and arrow shaped reflect ischemia. Elevated S-T segments reflect a current of injury from the nonfunctional tissue. An abnormal Q wave (exceeding 0.04 sec) reflects tissue necrosis (transmural).

There are other conditions that can mimic these ECG signs of infarction but do not evolve as does the myocardial infarction. Consequently it is important never to proceed on the ECG alone and never to make the diagnosis from a single tracing. One must see serial tracings in order to confirm an evolving pattern. This must then be evaluated in the context of the total clinical picture.

The evolving myocardial infarction initially has inverted T waves (ischemia), which give way to elevated S-T segments that are typically coved upward (injury current). As the myocardium heals, the elevated S-T segment resolves into inverted T waves. All this takes place over a period of two or three weeks. Finally, as the myocardium heals completely, except of course for the necrotic tissue, the T waves become upright. Necrosis is not reflected on the ECG unless it is transmural, that is, through and through the myocardial wall.

Once you know the evolving picture of myocardial infarction, it only remains for you to learn the reflecting leads in order to determine which cardiac surface(s) is involved.

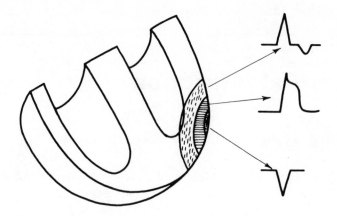

Fig. 17-1. Ischemia, injury, and necrosis as reflected in the ECG.

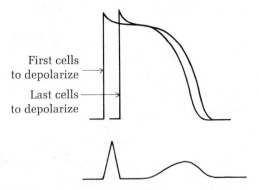

First cells
to depolarize

Last cells
to depolarize

Fig. 17-2. The normal S-T segment is isoelectric because during this time there is no difference in potential between the first and last cells to depolarize. (Modified from Surawicz, B., and Saito, S.: Am. J. Cardiol. **41:**943, 1978.)

Ischemia

Ischemia of tissue surrounding the infarct causes a reversal of the T wave. Because the depolarization process is changed as a result of local ischemia, the repolarization process is also altered. T wave inversion secondary to ischemia is typically symmetrical and arrow shaped.

Injury

Because of severe ischemia and lack of nutrients, the tissue immediately surrounding the center of the infarct is nonfunctional. It receives its blood supply from the collateral circulation. This is sufficient to keep it alive but insufficient to maintain membrane integrity, and a current of injury flows during repolarization (electrical systole) and/or during the resting phase (electrical diastole). The following discussion will acquaint you with the normal electrophysiology of the S-T segment and T wave, systolic and diastolic currents of injury, ST-T segment deviation not due to ischemia, epicardial versus endocardial injury patterns, reciprocal changes, and pathological Q waves. After this will be an explaination of the reflecting leads.

Normal S-T segment: electrophysiology

The S-T segment constitutes that portion of the ECG from the end of the QRS complex (J point) to the beginning of the T wave and corresponds to phase 2 of the action potential.

Remember that current flows in the myocardium when there is a difference in potential between myocardial cells. This is reflected by an appropriate displacement of the ECG stylus from the isoelectric line. In Fig. 17-2 note that the QRS complex is the result of a difference in electrical potential between the first and the last cells to depolarize (phase 0). Note also that during phase 2 of the action potential there is little difference in potential between the first and last cells to repolarize. This means that no current flows in the myocardium during this time—thus an isoelectric line (S-T segment).

Normal T wave: electrophysiology

During the rapid phase of repolarization (phase 3) there is a noticeable difference in potential between the first and the last cells to repolarize, since the last cells lag behind. This difference causes a current flow that produces the T wave. This fact is illustrated in Fig. 17-2. Note the space between the two repolarization lines in phase 3, indicating a difference in electrical potential and therefore current flow.

Currents of injury: systolic and diastolic

Myocardial ischemia may result in shortening and decreased amplitude of the action potential and/or a less negative resting membrane potential that is most likely due to a leakage of potassium from the injured cells.

Fig. 17-3 illustrates diagrammatically the currents of injury created by the differences in electrical potential between the first and the last myocardial cells to depolarize and repolarize.

Fig. 17-3, *A*, illustrates the difference in potential that can exist during repolarization (electrical systole) because some cells have action potentials of lesser amplitude and duration than normal. Note the space between the

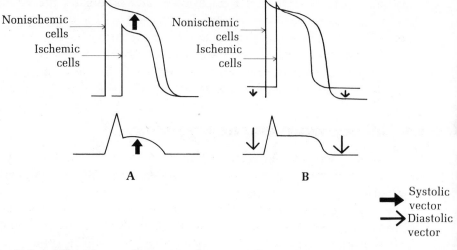

Fig. 17-3. A, Effect of a systolic current of injury on the ECG and action potential. One of the results of myocardial ischemia is to shorten the duration and decrease the amplitude of the action potential. Note that during electrical systole this creates a difference in potential between the first and the last cells to depolarize during the time that the S-T segment is inscribed. The resulting current displaces the S-T segment upward. **B,** Effect of a diastolic current of injury on the ECG and action potential. Another result of myocardial ischemia is a less negative resting membrane potential. Note that during electrical diastole this creates a difference in potential between the first and the last cells to depolarize during the T-Q segment. The resulting current displaces the baseline downward, producing an elevated S-T segment. (Modified from Surawicz, B., and Saito, S.: Am. J. Cardiol. **41:**943, 1978.

two action potentials during the time that the S-T segment is described on the ECG. The resulting current displaces the S-T segment upward.

Fig. 17-3, *B,* illustrates the difference in potential that can exist during phase 4 of the action potential (electrical diastole) because of differences in resting membrane potential. Note the space between the two action potentials during phase 4 (T-Q segment of the ECG). The resulting current displaces the baseline downward.

Both systolic and diastolic injury currents have the same end result, that is, S-T segment elevation.

S-T segment deviation and T wave changes not due to ischemia

When there is a delay in interventricular conduction time, there is a difference in potential between the first and last cells to depolarize during the entire repolarization process. Fig. 17-4, *A,* illustrates how there may be a deviation in the S-T segment accompanied by T wave changes secondary to interventricular conduction delay. Fig. 17-4, *B,* shows S-T segment deviation due to a shorter and steeper course of phase 2.

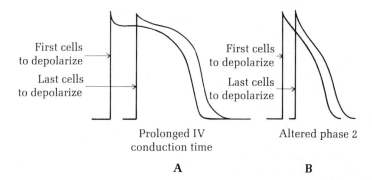

First cells
to depolarize

Last cells
to depolarize

First cells
to depolarize

Last cells
to depolarize

Prolonged IV
conduction time

Altered phase 2

A

B

Fig. 17-4. Altered action potentials of prolonged interventricular (IV) conduction time, digitalis effect, hypokalemia, or tachycardia. Note the difference in electrical potential between the first and last cells to depolarize during the entire repolarization process. (Modified from Surawicz, B., and Saito, S.: Am. J. Cardiol. **41**:943, 1978.)

Epicardial versus endocardial injury patterns

Fig. 17-5 illustrates the mechanism of S-T segment elevation in epicardial injury. Note that the systolic injury results in the S-T segment vector being directed anteriorly toward the reflecting lead, producing an elevation of the S-T segment. The diastolic injury current also produces this elevation because, being directed away from the reflecting lead, it produces a depression of the T-Q segment.

Fig. 17-6 illustrates the mechanism of S-T segment depression in endocardial injury. Note that the systolic injury results in the S-T segment vector being directed posteriorly, away from the reflecting lead, producing a depression of the S-T segment. The diastolic injury current compounds this depression because it is directed toward the reflecting lead, displacing the T-Q segment upward in the opposite direction from the S-T segment.

Reciprocal changes

When S-T segment elevation is found in leads facing one surface of the heart, S-T segment depression is often seen in the leads facing the opposite surface. For example, if the S-T segment is elevated in the inferior leads (II, III, and aV$_F$) due to a current of injury in the inferior wall of the heart, then some or all of the leads facing the superior lateral wall (precordial leads I and aV$_L$) may show the opposite effect, that is, S-T segment depression. This is illustrated in Fig. 17-7. Note that just as the S-T segment elevation is the result of an injury current flowing toward the inferior leads, the S-T segment depression is the result of this same current of injury flowing away from the leads on the opposite side of the heart.

Reciprocal changes may also be seen in the presence of abnormal Q

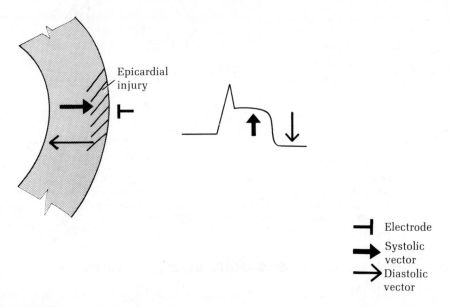

Fig. 17-5. Effect of systolic and diastolic injury vectors on the S-T segment because of epicardial injury. (Modified from Surawicz, B., and Saito, S.: Am. J. Cardiol. **41**:943, 1978.)

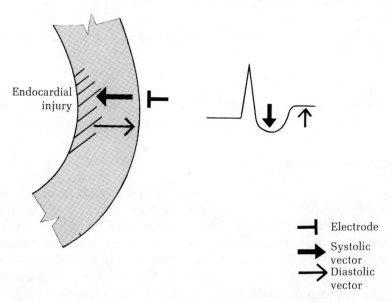

Fig. 17-6. Effect of systolic and diastolic injury vectors on the S-T segment because of endocardial injury. (Modified from Surawicz, B., and Saito, S.: Am. J. Cardiol. **41**:943, 1978.)

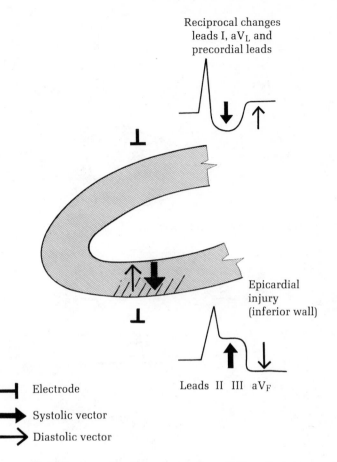

Reciprocal changes
leads I, aV$_L$ and
precordial leads

Epicardial
injury
(inferior wall)

Leads II III aV$_F$

Electrode

Systolic vector

Diastolic vector

Fig. 17-7. Reciprocal changes. Note the effect of systolic and diastolic injury vectors on the S-T segment in leads facing the wall opposite the injury.

waves and inverted T waves. In such cases the leads facing the opposite wall of the heart may record taller R and T waves.

Necrosis

Necrotic tissue has no polarity. This area of the infarct therefore acts as a window through which the electrode "sees" a current moving away from the infarcted area. This abnormally directed QRS vector causes a Q wave with a duration of more than 0.04 sec in leads facing the infarcted area (Fig. 17-8).

•   •   •

Myocardial necrosis, injury, and ischemia (Fig. 17-9) may be present at the same time, and the ECG manifestations of all three states may occur

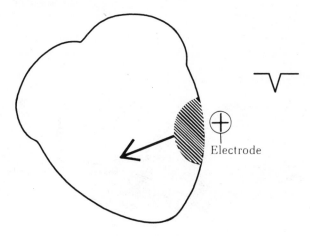

Fig. 17-8. Q wave is seen best in leads directly over the necrotic tissue.

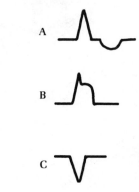

Fig. 17-9. A, Ischemia. **B,** Injury. **C,** Death.

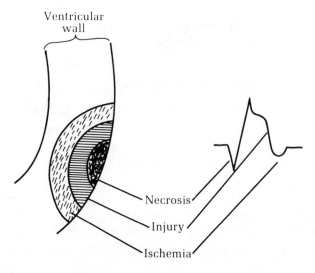

Fig. 17-10. All three grades of injury may be seen in one lead.

simultaneously (Fig. 17-10). The positive electrode closest to the infarcted area reflects the infarction most prominently.

Leads reflecting indicative changes

The surfaces of the heart and the leads that face them are illustrated in Fig. 17-11. Note that an inferior wall myocardial infarction is reflected in the inferior leads II, III, and aV_F. A high lateral wall myocardial infarction is seen only in the lateral leads I and aV_L. If it is lower on the lateral wall, it is also picked up by V_5 and V_6, which usually lie directly over the lateral wall near the apex. Leads V_1 to V_4 are directly over the anterior wall of the heart and reflect an myocardial infarction of this area.

Leads reflecting reciprocal changes

It is simplest to consider both the lateral and anterior walls as *superior*. It is then easy to understand why the reciprocal changes from an inferior wall myocardial infarction may show up in any of the precordial leads or in I and aV_L. Note in Fig. 17-11 that the leads reflecting the anterior wall and the lateral wall are both opposite the inferior wall. By the same token, an infarct of the anterior or lateral walls (both superior) may have reciprocal changes in the inferior leads (II, III, and aV_F). When looking at Fig. 17-11,

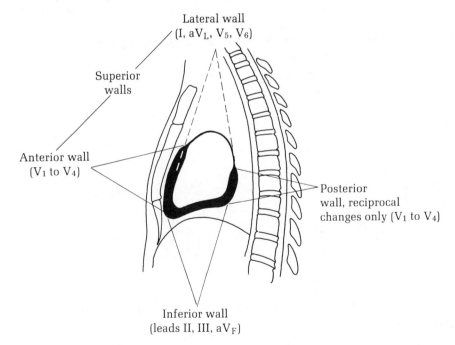

Fig. 17-11. Surfaces of the heart and the leads that face them.

if you can visualize the curve of the heart as it comes from the anterior wall to form the lateral wall, you will see that sometimes reciprocal changes from a lateral wall myocardial infarction show up in the precordial leads farthest to the right (V_1 and V_2) and vice versa.

Inferior wall myocardial infarction

Fig. 17-12 further illustrates the proximity of leads *II, III,* and *aV_F* to the inferior wall of the heart. These leads shall be referred to from now on simply as "the inferior leads." They are always evaluated as a group. When looking for an myocardial infarction in Fig. 17-13, *A,* look first at the inferior leads. Note the big elevated S-T segment and the pathological Q wave. These are signs of acute transmural myocardial infarction of the inferior wall. This surface is supplied by the posterior descending right coronary artery. If conduction problems occur with this patient, they will most probably be at the level of the AV node (Wenckebach). They will be ischemic rather than necrotic, since the area around the AV node is well supplied by the anterior descending left coronary artery.

Reciprocal changes are seen in V_1 to V_4. There is good R wave progression, and the small q wave in leads I and V_6 indicates normal septal activation.

Fig. 17-13, *B* was taken from the same patient 3 days later. Note in the inferior leads how the myocardial infarction has evolved. In the leads where acute injury was reflected, the S-T segment has come down, giving way to an inverted T wave (ischemia), which is typically symmetrical and arrow shaped. Reciprocal changes have disappeared, and QS complexes in the inferior leads produce left axis deviation (−60 degrees). Note that the left axis deviation of inferior wall myocardial infarction differs from that of

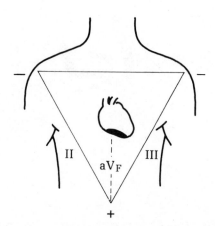

Fig. 17-12. Leads reflecting an inferior wall myocardial infarction.

anterior hemiblock in that the initial little r wave is absent in the inferior leads.

In Fig. 17-13, *B*, a change is seen in the leads reflecting the apical area (V₄ to V₆). The S-T segment is elevated, indicating an extension of the myocardial infarction to this surface. Note cessation of R wave progression.

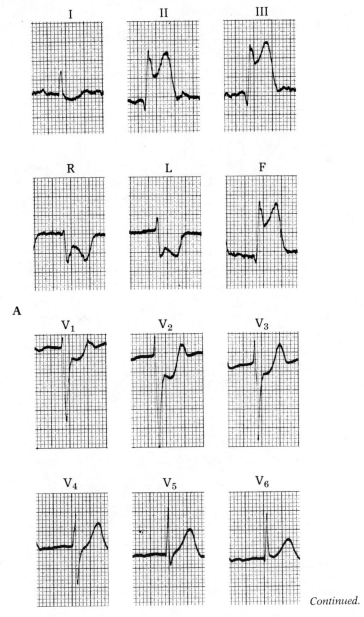

Continued.

Fig. 17-13. A, Acute evolving inferior wall myocardial infarction. Note the inferior leads. Reciprocal changes are seen in I, aV$_L$, and V₁ to V₃.

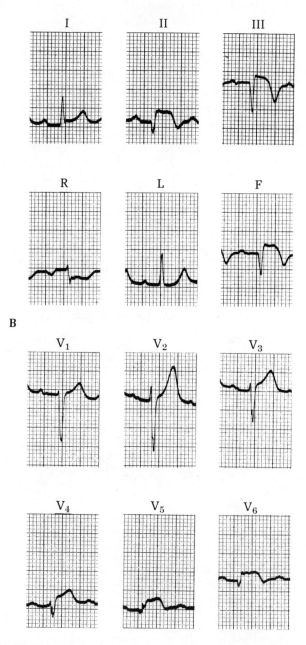

Fig. 17-13, cont'd. B, Same patient 3 days later. Note again the inferior leads. The acute injury pattern is resolving into a pattern of ischemia (inverted T waves). Note also that the pathological Q waves in **A** are now QS waves, producing a left axis deviation.

Anterior wall myocardial infarction

An infarction of the anterior wall of the heart results from an occlusion of the left anterior descending coronary artery or one of its branches. The conduction problems resulting from such an occlusion involve the bundle branches and are necrotic in nature.

Figs. 17-14 and 17-5 illustrate the further divisions of the anterior wall

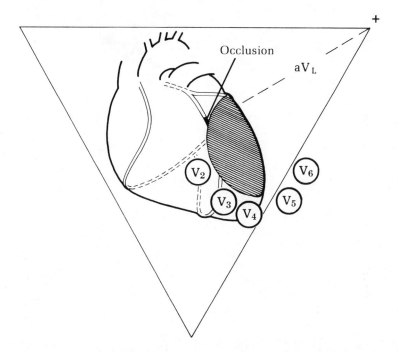

Fig. 17-14. Extensive anterior wall infarct.

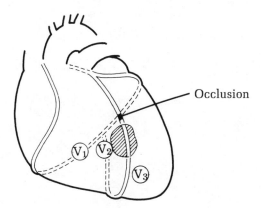

Fig. 17-15. Anteroseptal infarct.

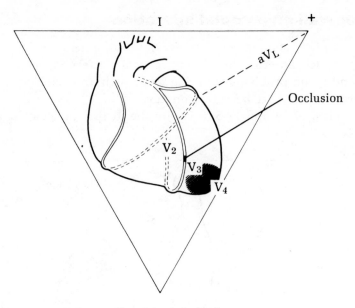

Fig. 17-16. Apical infarct.

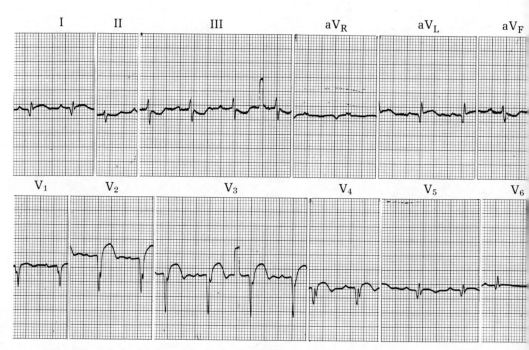

Fig. 17-17. Acute anterior wall myocardial infarction reflected in V_1 to V_4 with extension to the later wall (aV_L and I). Note the reciprocal changes in III and aV_F.

infarction into extensive anterior and anteroseptal. In Fig. 17-14 note that an extensive anterior wall infarction is reflected in all the precordial leads except perhaps V_1 and is seen in the lateral leads I and aV_L as well. In Fig. 17-15 note that an infarct confined to the anteroseptal region is seen in V_1 to V_3 and sometimes V_4. Fig. 17-16 illustrates the leads that may reflect any apical involvement, that is, V_2, to V_4. Changes may also show up in leads I and aV_L and V_5.

The 12 lead (V_6) in Fig. 17-17 reflects an acute, extensive anterior wall

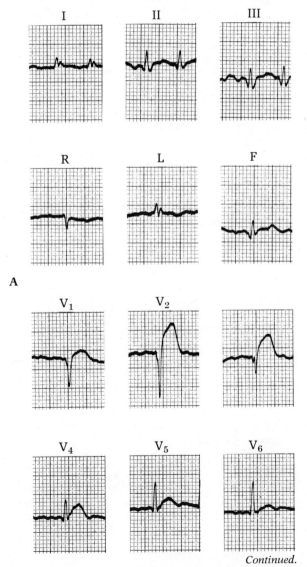

Continued.

Fig. 17-18. A, Acute anteroseptal myocardial infarction and old inferior wall myocardial infarction.

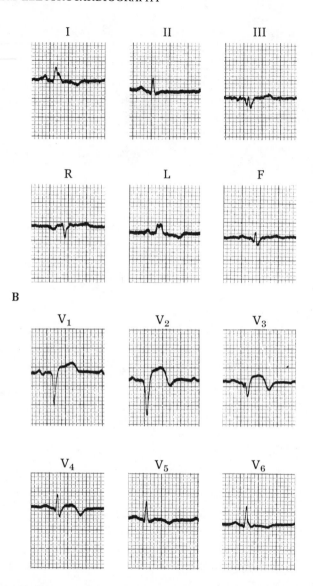

Fig. 17-18, cont'd. B, Same patient 1 week later. Note the evolvement of the anteroseptal pathology. The inferior leads remain the same.

myocardial infarction (sometimes called anterolateral). Note the loss of R wave progression in the precordial leads and the elevated S-T segments in these leads, with the typically coved upward appearance. Pathological Q waves and elevated S-T segments are also seen in leads *I* and *aV_L,* indicating an infarct such as is diagrammatically pictured in Fig. 17-14. Reciprocal changes are seen in leads *III* and *aV_F.*

An anteroseptal myocardial infarction is reflected in the 12 lead seen in

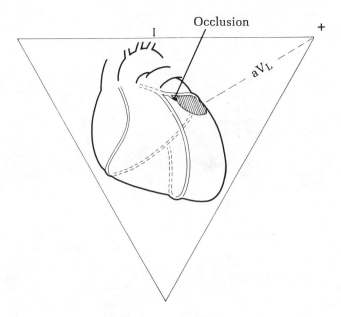

Fig. 17-19. Lateral wall infarct.

Fig. 17-18. Note the elevated, typically coved upward S-T segments in V_1 to V_4, with a loss of the R wave in V_1 to V_3. The pathological Q waves in the inferior leads are the remnants of an old inferior wall myocardial infarction. These do not evolve further as do the acute changes in the precordial leads. This fact is illustrated in Fig. 17-18, *B*, from the same patient 1 week later. Note that the Q waves in the inferior leads persist unchanged, while the acute anteroseptal pathology has evolved. The S-T segments have come down somewhat, and the T waves are beginning to invert.

Lateral wall infarction

If the infarct is confined to the lateral wall, changes are seen only in aV_L and lead I. This is diagrammatically illustrated in Fig. 17-19. The 12-lead ECG in Fig. 17-20 illustrates an acute, evolving lateral wall infarction. Note the S-T segment elevation in leads I and aV_L only. Reciprocal changes can be seen in the inferior leads and in V_2 to V_5.

Posterior wall infarction

Posterior wall infarction is caused by an occlusion of either the right coronary artery or a branch of the circumflex artery.

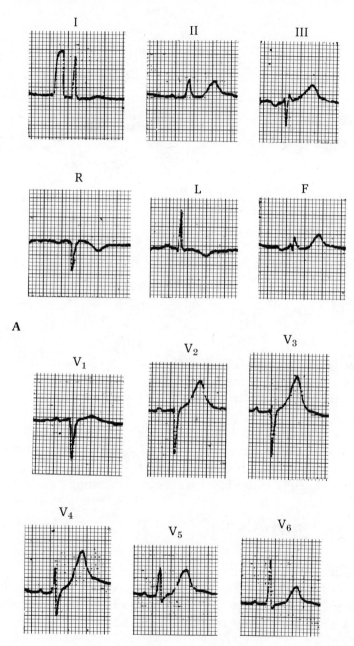

Fig. 17-20. A, Acute evolving lateral wall infarction. Note the S-T segment changes in I and aV$_L$.

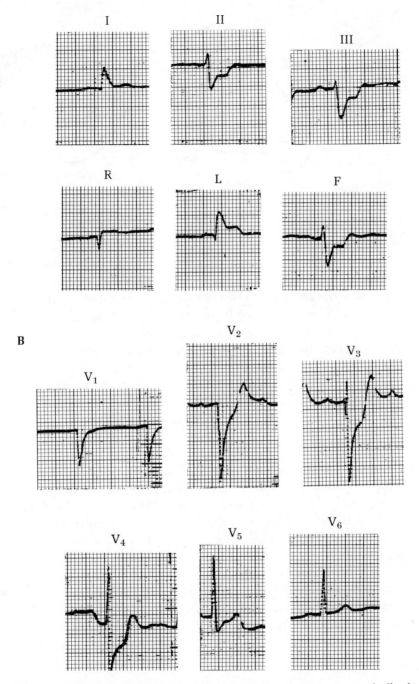

Fig. 17-20, cont'd. B, Same patient 2 days later. The S-T segment is now markedly elevated in I and aV$_L$. There are reciprocal changes in the inferior lead and in V$_2$ to V$_5$.

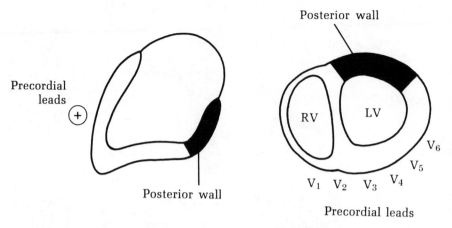

Fig. 17-21. Posterior wall infarction.

Because there are no leads directly over true *posterior wall*, changes are reflected in the leads on the opposite wall. These are reciprocal changes only. This is illustrated in Fig. 17-21. Therefore, instead of an abnormal Q wave, there is a tall, broad initial R. Instead of an S-T segment elevation due to an injury current traveling away from the electrode, there is an S-T segment depression due to an injury current traveling toward the electrode. The T wave is upright rather than inverted. The 12-lead ECG in Fig. 17-22 illustrates a true posterior myocardial infarction. Note the tall R wave in V_1 to V_4 and the reciprocal ST-T wave changes.

Stages of recovery

During the acute phases of infarction, when there is a greater amount of nonfunctional and necrotic tissue, S-T segment displacements and QRS changes are seen. As the nonfunctional tissue either dies or becomes functional again, the S-T segment displacements disappear and are replaced by inverted T waves, an indication of secondary ischemia (the nonfunctional tissue in becoming functional is still ischemic).

These processes take anywhere from several days to 3 weeks. As healing progresses, the Q wave regresses. In most cases it persists permanently. However, in some cases when the dead tissue becomes fibrosed and turns to scar tissue, the area may be so small that it is not demonstrated on the ECG.

Pericarditis

Since deviation of the S-T segment and inversion of the T wave are also the features of pericarditis, I have included pericarditis in this chapter.

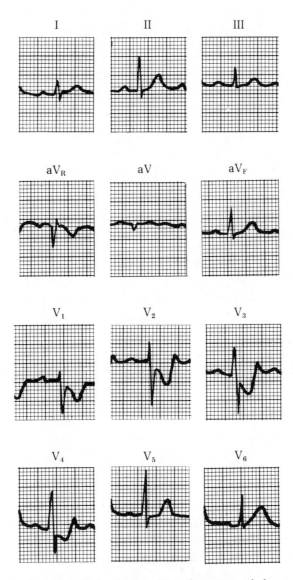

Fig. 17-22. True posterior myocardial infarction. Note the reciprocal changes in V_1 to V_4, that is, tall R waves, depressed S-T segments, and tall T waves in V_2 to V_4. (From Conover, M.: Cardiac arrhythmias exercises in pattern interpretation, ed. 2, St. Louis, 1978, The C. V. Mosby Co.)

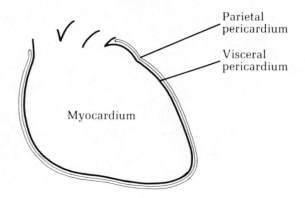

Fig. 17-23. Pericardium.

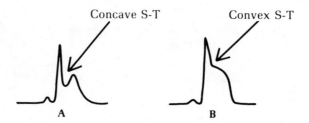

Fig. 17-24. A, Pericarditis. **B**, Myocardial infarction.

ANATOMICAL ASPECTS

The heart is enveloped in two membranes, the *visceral* and the *parietal pericardium* (Fig. 17-23). Inflammation of either one or both of these membranes is called pericarditis.

ELECTROPHYSIOLOGY

The epicardial surface beneath the inflamed area is unable to polarize. There is therefore an injury current (elevated S-T segment) in leads reflecting the involved area. As the disease becomes less acute, the upward displacement of the S-T segment disappears, returning to the isoelectric line or below it, and the T wave becomes inverted. The T wave changes occur during the subacute stage and are attributed to delayed repolarization of the epicardium, which is usually the first to repolarize.

ECG changes

1. *S-T segment:* In myocardial infarction there is, in most cases, reciprocal S-T segment depression. For example, if there is elevation of the S-T seg-

ment in a lead over the infarction, there will be a reciprocal depression of the S-T segment in a lead over the opposite surface of the heart. In acute pericarditis this reciprocal S-T depression rarely occurs. Rather, because of the diffuse nature of pericarditis, the S-T segment elevation is seen in all leads reflecting epicardial potentials. The S-T segment also looks different in pericarditis, taking a concave form as opposed to the convex form seen in myocardial infarction (Fig. 17-24).

2. *T wave:* In pericarditis the T wave may be inverted in all three standard leads (I, II, and III). This is significant and seldom occurs in myocardial infarction. Usually in pericarditis the T wave inversion occurs in leads I and II.

3. *Q waves:* The characteristic Q waves of myocardial infarction do not occur in pericarditis.

Selected readings

Marriott, H. J. L.: Practical electrocardiography, ed. 6, Baltimore, 1977, The Williams & Wilkins Co.

Schamroth, L.: An introduction to electrocardiography, Philadelphia, 1976, Blackwell Scientific Publications.

Surawicz, B., and Saito, S.: Exercise testing for detection of myocardial ischemia in patients with abnormal electrocardiograms at rest, Am. J. Cardiol. **41:**943, 1978.

CHAPTER 18

Drugs and electrolytes and their effect on the ECG

Sympathetic nervous system

The sympathetic nerve (Fig. 18-1) is composed of a *preganglionic fiber*, where the hormone *acetylcholine* is released; a cholinergic receptor (receiver of acetyl*choline*); a *postganglionic fiber*, where the hormone *norepinephrine* is released; and an *adrenergic receptor* (receiver of norepinephrine).

Norepinephrine is the neurotransmitter of sympathetic adrenergic nerves. The adrenergic receptor is the site on the muscle or gland where norepinephrine acts. It is also the site of action of epinephrine (adrenal medullary hormone) and adrenergic drugs (related structurally to endogenous catecholamines).

In 1948 Ahlquist[1] postulated that there are at least two different kinds of adrenergic receptor, which he named *alpha* and *beta*. When stimulated, these receptors trigger a characteristic response of a muscle or gland. The response mediated through the alpha receptors is vasoconstriction; through the beta receptors it is cardiac stimulation and vasodilatation. Beta receptors have been further separated into *beta*$_1$, for the heart, and *beta*$_2$, for peripheral vasculature and the bronchioles.[2,3]

All blood vessels have both alpha and beta receptors, although one or the other may dominate in certain areas. For example, alpha receptors dominate in the skin and kidneys, while beta receptors dominate in the vascular beds of skeletal muscle. Both receptors are active in coronary, visceral, and connective tissue.

ARRHYTHMIAS RESULTING FROM SYMPATHETIC STIMULATION

Sinus tachycardia is the normal response of the heart to sympathetic activity. Latent pacemaker sites also increase their inherent rate, but this is normally dominated by the sinus tachycardia and thus is not manifest unless the sinus tachycardia does not occur. Such arrhythmias are the result of enhanced automaticity due to a more rapid deactivation of the slow outward potassium current.

Sympathetic stimulation may also result in arrhythmias due to reentry, both focal and circus.[4]

TERMINOLOGY

adrenergic Refers to the receptors (alpha and beta) for norepinephrine or the sympathetic nerve.

adrenergic drugs Act at this effector site.

alpha and beta receptors Specific receptive sites within the effector cell or end organ.

catecholamines A particular group of vasoactive sympathetic endogenous mediators; dopamine, norepinephrine, and epinephrine are included in this category.

chronotropic effect Refers to heart rate and may be either positive or negative.

dromotropic Refers to a conduction velocity.

inotropic effect Refers to myocardial contractility and may be either positive or negative.

norepinephrine Mediator of the sympathetic nerve.

sympatholytic drugs (Gr. lytikos = dissolving) Block the effects of the sympathetic nervous system at the nerve terminal or at the receptor site (alpha or beta).

sympathomimetic drugs (mimetic = mimic) Mimic the effects of stimuli to the sympathetic nervous system by stimulating the nerve ending.

SYMPATHOMIMETIC DRUGS
(STIMULANTS OF THE SYMPATHETIC NERVOUS SYSTEM)

The action of the sympathetic nervous system can be enhanced at the nerve terminal, where norepinephrine is released, and at the alpha or beta adrenergic receptor sites on the effector cell (Fig. 18-1).

Some clinically useful sympathomimetic drugs follow.

Epinephrine (Adrenaline) is the most potent sympathomimetic because of its strong mediation through both alpha and beta receptors. The results of an intravenous infusion of epinephrine depend on the clinical setting. It may produce tachycardia, increase in pulse pressure, increase in cardiac output, decrease in total peripheral resistance, decrease in diastolic pressure, and intense cutaneous and renal vasoconstriction.[5] It produces gangrene if injected into areas with only alpha receptors.

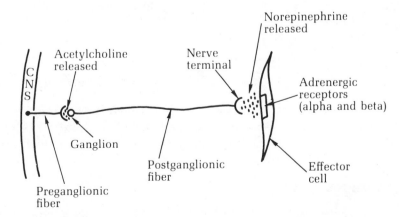

Fig. 18-1. Sympathetic nerve. *CNS*, Central nervous system.

Norepinephrine (or *levarterenol, Levophed*) has predominately alpha effects when administered exogenously,[5] whereas endogenous norepinephrine, being the neurotransmitter of the sympathetic nervous system, acts through both alpha and beta receptors. Because of its strong alpha effects, norepinephrine can be administered only intravenously. It produces an increase in peripheral vascular resistance and an increase in diastolic pressure. Bradycardia is the response to an increase in mean arterial pressure. Norepinephrine also causes a marked decrease in renal blood flow.

Infiltration of the drug into the perivenous tissue results in tissue necrosis, which is counteracted by an alpha blocking agent (phentolamine).

Phenylephrine (Neo-Synephrine) has alpha effects only, causing peripheral vasoconstriction. If there is an increase in mean arterial pressure, bradycardia results. This drug may be administered subcutaneously, intramuscularly, or intravenously.

Methoxamine (Vasoxyl) has actions similar to those of phenylephrine.

Isoproterenol (Isuprel) has beta effects only, with positive inotropic, chronotropic, and dromotropic effects, as well as vasodilatation that is greatest in skeletal muscle and least in the kidney.

Dopamine (Intropin) acts on the beta receptors of the heart. Its effect on renal circulation is dose related and reflects its action on dopaminergic receptors. In low and moderate doses it increases renal blood flow, whereas in high doses it produces renal vasoconstriction.[3]

Dobutamine (Dobutrex), a synthetic derivative of isoproterenol, acts directly on the beta receptors of the heart, as does dopamine. However, unlike dopamine, it does not cause norepinephrine to be released from the nerve endings. It increases myocardial contractility but has less effect on the beta receptors in the arterioles and lungs than do other sympathomimetics.[6]

Terbutaline (Bricanyl) acts primarily on the beta receptors of smooth muscle with only a slight effect on the heart, making it useful in the treatment of bronchial asthma.

Mephentermine (Wyamine) acts indirectly by displacing the norepinephrine stored in the nerve ends to produce cardiac stimulation and vasoconstriction.

Metaraminol (Aramine) acts indirectly by replacing the norepinephrine stored in the nerve ends and directly through alpha receptors to produce vasopressor effects. Because this drug enters the storage mechanism at the nerve ends, there is an impairment in nerve function when long-term infusion is discontinued.

NERVE TERMINAL STIMULANTS

The nerve terminal stimulants are drugs that cause norepinephrine to be released from the nerve ending, and consequently they have both alpha and beta effects. Examples are tyramine and ephedrine.

SYMPATHOLYTIC DRUGS (ANTAGONISTS OF THE SYMPATHETIC NERVOUS SYSTEM)

The action of the sympathetic nervous system can be blocked at three places (Fig. 18-1):

1. The adrenergic receptor (alpha or beta), where norepinephrine is received
2. The nerve terminal, where norepinephrine is released
3. The ganglion

Adrenergic blocking agents

Adrenergic blocking agents act mainly by competing with catecholamines for positions on the receptor site. Such drugs are called *competitive blockers*. Phentolamine (Regitine) and tolazoline (Priscoline) are alpha competitive blockers; propranolol (Inderal) is a beta competitive blocker. Phenoxybenzamine (Dibenzyline) is a noncompetitive alpha blocker in that it changes the alpha receptor chemically.

Alpha adrenergic blocking agents. Alpha-adrenergic blocking agents cause vascular dilatation. Thus they induce a reduction in peripheral resistance and venous return and elicit fainting and compensatory tachycardia as soon as the individual stands up unless neurogenic vasoconstriction is present.

Tolazoline and *phentolamine* are short-acting competitive alpha blockers with a histamine-like action that complicates their effect. Tolazoline is also a beta stimulant and a muscarinic drug useful in peripheral vascular disease. Phentolamine has been used to diagnose pheochromocytoma, to treat accidental tissue infiltration by norepinephrine or dopamine, and to treat hypovolemic shock.[7]

Phenoxybenzamine has been used in peripheral vascular disease, treatment of pheochromocytoma, and hypovolemic shock.[7]

Beta adrenergic blocking agents. The chief cardiovascular effect of beta blockade is bradycardia, resulting from removal of sympathetic control of the heart.

Propranolol and metoprolol[5] are the only beta blockers in use in the United States. Practolol is widely used in Europe. Other beta blockers are sotalol, alprenolol, oxprenolol, pindolol, timolol, and atenolol.[7,8]

ANTIARRHYTHMIC EFFECT OF BETA BLOCKADE. Use of beta blockade for arrhythmias may be precluded because of the negative inotropic, chronotropic, and dromotropic effects and because of the development of hypotension and bronchospasm.

Long-term *propranolol* has been effective in the following:

1. Atrial and ventricular arrhythmias due to excessive sympathetic activity
2. Digitalis-induced atrial and ventricular arrhythmias, although the

presence of AV block would contraindicate the use of propranolol

3. Combination with an antiarrhythmic agent (quinidine or procainamide) to prevent the recurrence of atrial fibrillation after direct current (DC) cardioversion[9]

Metoprolol is a cardioselective beta blocker with very little effect on the beta receptors of the arterioles and lungs.[10,11]

Nerve terminal blocking agents

Nerve terminal blocking agents interfere with sympathetic nervous system activity by decreasing the available norepinephrine, thereby inhibiting both alpha and beta responses. This is accomplished by the following:

1. Preventing the release of norepinephrine (bretylium tosylate)
2. Inhibiting the synthesis of norepinephrine (methyltyrosine)
3. Depleting the nerve ending of norepinephrine (reserpine and guanethidine)

Ganglionic blocking agents

Both the sympathetic and parasympathetic systems are affected by these drugs, since both systems have ganglia. They cause orthostatic hypotension, reduced venous return, and reduced peripheral resistance.

Parasympathetic nervous system

The parasympathetic nerve is composed of a *preganglionic fiber*, where acetylcholine is released; a cholinergic receptor, where acetylcholine is

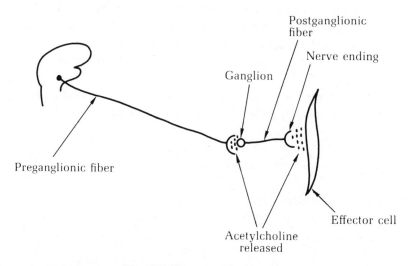

Fig. 18-2. Parasympathetic nerve.

received; a *postganglionic fiber*, where acetylcholine is again released; and cholinergic receptors located on the *effector cell* (end organ) (Fig. 18-2).

PARASYMPATHETIC FUNCTION COMPARED TO SYMPATHETIC FUNCTION

The vagus nerve supplies the parasympathetic innervation to the heart, mainly the atria. Thus these nerves (vagi) control the supraventricular functions of heart rate and AV conduction.

Conversely, the ventricles are rich in sympathetic nerve innervation and poor in vagus innervation. Thus it is that the sympathetic nerves control ventricular function via the beta receptors. Therefore drugs blocking or stimulating the vagus nerve exert their effect mostly on the sinus and AV nodes, enhancing or blocking rate and conduction. For example, atropine blocks the effects of the vagus nerve and has little effect on ventricular function.

By the same token, drugs blocking or stimulating the sympathetic nervous system affect the ventricles. For example, propranolol, a beta adrenergic blocking agent, markedly affects ventricular contractility and has only a moderate effect on the sinus or AV nodes.

TERMINOLOGY

acetylcholine Mediator of the parasympathetic nerve.
cholinergic Refers to the receptors for acetylcholine or the parasympathomimetic drugs; these receptors are located in the ganglion and in the effector cell.
cholinesterase An enzyme in the cholinergic receptors that is responsible for the breakdown or inactivation of acetylcholine.
cholinesterase inhibitors Enhance the effects of the parasympathetic nervous system by slowing the inactivation of acetylcholine, thus allowing the characteristic actions of the parasympathetic nervous system to proceed in an intensified manner; physostigmine (eserine), neostigmine, and edrophonium chloride are examples.
parasympatholytic drugs (Gr. lytikos = dissolving) Block or dissolve the effects of the parasympathetic nervous system.
parasympathomimetic drugs (mimetic = mimic) Mimic the effects of stimuli to the parasympathetic nervous system.

ACETYLCHOLINE

As mediator of the parasympathetic nerve, acetylcholine has a negative chronotropic effect, decreasing the rate of the sinus node. It causes vasodilatation, which in turn elicits a reflex increase of sympathetic activity. Thus there is an increase in the heart rate and cardiac output as a compensatory activity.

CHOLINERGIC BLOCKING DRUGS

Cholinergic blocking drugs act by blocking the action of acetylcholine at the effector cell.

Atropine is this type of drug and causes an increase in heart rate and AV conduction. The site of the action of atropine is directly on the *effector cells* and not on the *nerve endings* (Fig. 18-2). There it blocks the action of acetylcholine but not its liberation, thus reversing all the effects of parasympathetic nervous stimulation. The heart rate is stimulated as a result of the blockage of vagal effects on the sinus node.

Antiarrhythmic drugs

Antiarrhythmic drugs achieve their desired effect through the following electrophysiological mechanisms:
1. Depressing diastolic depolarization (phase 4) through an alteration of membrane permeability to potassium, sodium (quinidine, lidocaine, procainamide, and propranolol), and calcium (verapamil).
2. Enhancing conduction velocity through an increase in the rate of rise of phase 0 (phenytoin) or through an increase in the resting membrane potential (bretylium)
3. Further depressing conduction velocity through a lowering of the resting membrane potential and a decrease in the rate of rise of phase 0 (quinidine, procainamide, and propranolol)

Prominent adverse drug reactions are found in Table 3.

Arrhythmias occurring during the first few minutes after coronary occlusion are thought to be the result of a reentry mechanism, whereas arrhythmias developing in the late ischemic period are thought to be the result of enhanced automaticity. Before antiarrhythmics are discussed, it should be mentioned that some investigators have found in their experiments on the canine heart that neither lidocaine nor procainamide prevents the very early arrhythmias of acute ischemia and that propranolol does so mainly by a reduction of heart rate. It has been shown in the clinical setting that acute myocardial infarction patients with sinus bradycardia have a lower mortality than those with sinus tachycardia. Heart rate should therefore be taken into consideration in the treatment of arrhythmias and the use of antiarrhythmic drugs.

It should also be noted that the effects of many antiarrhythmic drugs on the cellular membrane can be completely nullified by hypokalemia.

LIDOCAINE

Lidocaine was first used as a cardiac antiarrhythmic in 1950.[12] Since then it has become the most widely used antiarrhythmic drug in the treatment and prevention of ventricular ectopics in acute myocardial infarction. It is generally concluded that lidocaine is ineffective in suppressing most atrial arrhythmias.

The mechanism of action of lidocaine is similar to that of procainamide

Table 3. Prominent adverse drug reactions with ten
antiarrhythmic agents*

	Cardiovascular	Gastrointestinal	Central nervous system	Other
Quinidine	Prolong Q-T IVCD, HB Hypotension VPBs, VF	A/N/V Diarrhea Cramps	Auditory and visual disturbances	"Syncope" (VF) Thrombocytopenia Respiratory arrest
Procainamide	IVCD, HB Hypotension VPBs	A/N/V Diarrhea	Hallucinations	Fever, rash L.E. syndrome Agranulocytosis
Lidocaine	IVCD, HB Hypotension	Nausea	Sedation Somnolence Confusion Respiratory arrest	Tinnitus Paresthesias
Phenytoin	Hypotension Asystolic arrest	Vomiting Gastritis	Ataxia Nystagmus	Pseudolymphoma Megaloblastic anemia Hepatitis
Propranolol	CHF, HB Sinus bradycardia Hypotension	Nausea Diarrhea	Depression Dreams	Fatigue Hypoglycemia Asthma
Bretylium	Sinus bradycardia Hypotension	Nausea Diarrhea	Sedation	Nasal stuffiness Parotitis Urinary retention
Atropine	Sinus tachycardia	Dry mouth Constipation	Confusion Delirium	Flushing Urinary retention Glaucoma
Digitalis	Arrhythmias	A/N/V Diarrhea	Delirium Scotomas	Gynecomastia
Potassium	Bradycardia IVCD, HB Cardiac arrest	Anorexia Gastritis	N-M irrita- bility	Phlebitis
Isoproterenol	Tachycardia Hypotension VPBs, VF Angina pectoris	Nausea	Tremor	Nervousness

*From Moss, A., and Patton, R.: Antiarrhythmic agents, Springfield, Ill., 1973, Charles C
Thomas, Publisher.
A/N/V = anorexia, nausea, vomiting; CHF = congestive heart failure; HB = heart block;
IVCD = intraventricular conduction disturbance; VF = ventricular fibrillation; VPBs = ven-
tricular premature beats.

RECOMMENDATIONS FOR LIDOCAINE PROPHYLAXIS*

1. *Loading dose* (objective to administer 200 mg in 10 to 20 minutes)
   a. 100 mg given over a 2-minute period at 10-minute intervals
      or
   b. 50 mg in 1 minute, given four times, 5 minutes apart
      or
   c. 20 mg/min infused for 10 minutes
2. *Continuous administration* (infusion-regulating device necessary)
   a. 2 to 4 mg/min for 24 to 30 hours (average, 3 mg/min)
3. *To raise plasma concentration acutely* (for breakthrough ventricular arrhythmias)
   a. 50 mg bolus over 1 minute with simultaneous increase in infusion rate to no more than 5 mg/min
4. *To discontinue drug:* Stop intravenous infusion immediately
5. *In shock, heart failure, hepatocellular liver disease and in patients over 70 years old*
   a. Reduce doses by half for loading and infusion rate
   b. Measure serum concentrations frequently

---

*Modified from Harrison, D.C.: Should lidocaine be administered routinely to all patients after acute myocardial infarction? Circulation **58**:583, 1978. By permission of the American Heart Association, Inc.

RECOMMENDATIONS FOR LIDOCAINE AND PROCAINAMIDE WHEN ACUTE MYOCARDIAL INFARCTION IS SUSPECTED[16,19,20]

1. *All patients suspected of having acute MI:* 75 mg bolus of lidocaine (50 mg/min), followed by a 2 mg/min infusion controlled by an infusion pump; done in the emergency room
2. *Coronary care unit (CCU):*
   a. Transport to CCU with infusion pump, monitor, and defibrillator
   b. In CCU, an additional 50 mg bolus of lidocaine
3. *If PVCs continue:* Lidocaine, 50 mg bolus every 5 minutes if necessary to a total of 225 mg, increasing the infusion by 1 mg/min after each bolus to a maximum of 4 mg/min
4. *If ventricular ectopics not controlled:* Give procainamide, 100 mg bolus (over a 3-min period), every 5 minutes as necessary to a total of 1 g, beginning infusion(s) according to the number of boluses necessary:
   - 1-2 boluses = 2 mg/min
   - 3-4 boluses = 3 mg/min
   - 5-6 boluses = 4 mg/min
   - 7-8 boluses = 5 mg/min
   - over 8 boluses = 6 mg/min
5. *For breakthrough arrhythmias after stability:* Lidocaine, 25 to 50 mg bolus, or procainamide, 50 to 100 mg bolus, with the continuous infusion increased 1 mg/min (unless the maximum infusion rate has been reached)
6. *If procainamide alone fails:* Both lidocaine and procainamide used together

and quinidine, in that it causes conduction delay in severely depressed cells, with little or no effect on normal or moderately depressed cells.[13,14] It thus abolishes arrhythmias sustained by circus reentry by causing a two-way block in the depressed fibers.

Lidocaine also abolishes the arrhythmias due to focal reentry by the following mechanism: In infarcted myocardium the effective refractory period shortens, causing a current flow from the normal to the ischemic zone. Lidocaine prolongs the effective refractory period of the infarcted tissue but not of the normal tissue, decreasing the likelihood of such depolarizing currents.[13]

Lidocaine also depresses automaticity. Because this is accomplished in latent pacemaker cells at concentrations that do not suppress the sinus node, lidocaine restores the sinus node as the dominant pacemaker.[15]

Therapeutic dosage

Therapeutic plasma concentrations of lidocaine decline within minutes after a single bolus injection. A single loading dose is therefore unsatisfactory. The loading dose must be combined with an infusion to raise the plasma concentration to an antiarrhythmic level (1.4 to 6 μg/ml). One program for the administration of lidocaine is recommended on p. 228.

Some authorities recommend that lidocaine should be routinely administered to all patients with acute myocardial infarction[16,17] for the purpose of preventing primary ventricular fibrillation and because warning arrhythmias are frequently not detected. Additionally, the danger of toxicity is minimized because the pharmacokinetics of lidocaine are now well understood.[18] A regimen successfully used by one group for all patients suspected of having myocardial infarction is represented on p. 228.

Lidocaine is metabolized by the liver, its clearance approaching hepatic blood flow. With normal hepatic blood flow and function, plasma clearance is about 10 ml/kg/min.[18] Any condition that alters hepatic function or decreases blood flow causes an increase in plasma clearance time. Thus in shock, heart failure, hepatocellular liver disease, and patients over 70 years old, the loading doses and infusion rate should be reduced by one half.[17] (Although in liver disease, since the initial volume of distribution is little changed, the loading dose initially given need not be altered.[18])

Toxicity

Lidocaine toxicity is rare when rational programs for administration are used. Toxic plasma levels (6 μg/ml) produce symptoms reflective of central nervous system and/or cardiovascular involvement. Such reactions may be excitatory and/or depressant, characterized by nervousness, dizziness, blurred vision, and tremors, and followed by drowsiness and convulsions.

A small percentage of patients experience minor and *transient* central nervous system side effects when plasma levels are in the therapeutic range. Such side effects include tingling and numbness of the lips and fingers, a change in hearing perception, a buzzing sound, and a feeling of drowsiness.[16]

PROCAINAMIDE AND QUINIDINE

Procainamide and quinidine are useful for both atrial and ventricular arrhythmias. Their antiarrhythmic properties are due to the following mechanisms:

1. Both drugs have an antifibrillatory action because they increase the effective refractory period.
2. Atrial fibrillation and flutter may be terminated because these drugs slow the rate of repolarization and thus may abolish the wave fronts sustaining such arrhythmias.
3. Reentrant PVCs may be abolished because conduction is slowed and then blocked through the reentrant pathway.
4. Arrhythmias due to enhanced automaticity may be abolished because both drugs depress the slope of phase 4.[21] However, it has been shown that procainamide has no effect on slow channel automaticity.[22] Thus procainamide is not used to treat the PVCs that result from digitalis toxicity.
5. AV nodal reentrant tachycardia may be abolished because conduction is depressed in the retrograde AV nodal fast pathway by procainamide.[23]
6. Both drugs may also be effective in the treatment of the reentrant tachycardia of WPW syndrome because they prolong the effective refractory period of the accessory pathway. These drugs may also be used to decrease the ventricular rates when atrial fibrillation and flutter complicate this syndrome.

Procainamide

Therapeutic dosage and administration.[23,24] Procainamide is eliminated equally by the kidneys and the liver, with an average half-life for elimination of 3 to 4 hours in the normal adult. The therapeutic plasma level is from 3 to 10 μg/ml. In cardiac and renal failure dosage should be reduced by 30% to 50%.

INTRAVENOUS. Procainamide is administered in 100 mg doses intravenously at 5-minute intervals until either 1 g has been given, a therapeutic effect has been achieved, or toxic effects have appeared. Administration of the drug at 5-minute intervals is necessary because the plasma level falls rapidly after each injection.

With the first intravenous injection an infusion is started. The infusion rate should be from 2 to 4 mg/min (20 to 80 μg/kg/min).

ORAL. The first oral dose should not be administered until 4 hours after the infusion has been discontinued to avoid toxic plasma levels.

Procainamide is given orally in doses of approximately 50 mg/kg/24 hr (3.5 g). Because plasma levels vary from patient to patient, individual titration is necessary. A 3-hour dosing interval avoids the excessive peaks and troughs that result from the rapid fall in plasma level 1 to 2 hours after each dose.

Antiarrhythmic metabolite: *N*-acetyl procainamide. *N*-Acetyl procainamide is the major metabolite of procainamide. It has antiarrhythmic properties of its own, is almost entirely eliminated by the kidneys, and is not cleared as fast as procainamide. Thus, the total concentration of antiarrhythmics in the blood may be more than just the level of procainamide. Because this metabolite is eliminated through the kidneys, in renal failure the plasma levels of both procainamide and *N*-acetyl procainamide should be monitored.

Side effects. Studies have shown that when procainamide is taken for longer than 3 months, a syndrome resembling systemic lupus erythematosus will occur in approximately 40% of patients, with symptoms reversing on termination of the drug. Other undesirable side effects include anorexia, nausea, vomiting, diarrhea, flushing, skin rashes, chills, fever, mental depression, psychosis, and convulsions.

Quinidine

Therapeutic dosage and administration. Quinidine is eliminated almost entirely by metabolism, only 17% being excreted unchanged in the urine.[21] Thus the dosage should be reduced in patients with kidney failure. Therapeutic plasma level is from 2 to 6 μg/ml,[24] and plasma monitoring is highly desirable because of the toxic potential and variable pharmacokinetics of quinidine.

Quinidine is usually given orally with an initial total daily dose of 600 to 900 mg, which varies from individual to individual. Since quinidine gluconate is less rapidly absorbed than quinidine sulfate, it can be given less frequently (quinidine gluconate, every 8 to 12 hours; quinidine sulfate, every 6 to 8 hours.[18,25]).

Phenobarbital or phenytoin increases the elimination of quinidine.[26]

Side effects.[24] The most commonly cited toxic manifestation of oral quinidine administration is diarrhea. Nausea and vomiting occur less frequently.

An early sign of cardiovascular toxicity is Q-T prolongation, although this interval may also be prolonged in the absence of toxicity. QRS prolongation is a major sign of toxicity and is reflective of a decreased conduction velocity.

Quinidine may also cause cinchonism, thrombocytopenia (due to platelet lysis), and rarely anaphylactic reactions.

If the patient is taking oral anticoagulants, the quinidine interaction may cause unexpected bleeding.

Treatment of toxicity[24]

1. *Sodium lactate intravenously* lowers the plasma potassium level and changes the plasma pH. Toxic effects are diminished because increased potassium concentrations intensify the effects of quinidine and procainamide on the heart and because the change in pH increases the binding of quinidine to albumin.
2. *Beta-adrenergic amines* diminish the effect of quinidine and procainamide on the heart and counteract their negative inotropic effects.

PHENYTOIN (DILANTIN)

Phenytoin is highly effective against atrial and ventricular arrhythmias resulting from digitalis toxicity. It has little effect on atrial fibrillation, atrial flutter, or recurrent ventricular tachycardia.

Recently El-Sherif and Lazzara[27] have described the mechanism of action of phenytoin and have found that, like lidocaine, it selectively depresses conduction in ischemic fibers, with no effect on normal fibers. It thus abolishes arrhythmias sustained by a reentrant pathway by producing a complete block in the depressed fibers.[28]

Therapeutic dosage and administration

Phenytoin is eliminated entirely by metabolism. The therapeutic plasma level is from 10 to 20 μg/ml. Because this drug has an approximate half-life of 22 hours, 3 to 4 days are required to reach a steady plasma level. Usually 750 to 1000 mg in divided doses are given over the first 24 hours for loading. This is followed by a daily dose of 300 to 400 mg. Phenytoin may be administered intravenously or orally. Intramuscular injections can cause necrosis of the tissue. Plasma level monitoring is advised because the metabolism of phenytoin becomes saturated with a therapeutic range of concentrations, which varies from patient to patient.

When phenytoin is administered intravenously, small 50- to 100-mg injections should be given over 5 to 10 minutes (to avoid hypotension or arrhythmias) until toxicity occurs, the arrhythmia is controlled, or 1000 mg has been given.[18]

Orally phenytoin can be given with an initial dose of 300 mg, followed by 200 mg doses every 2 to 3 hours up to toxicity or a total of 900 to 1100 mg.[18]

Side effects

Rapid intravenous infusion of phenytoin may produce hypotension. The signs of central nervous system toxicity are drowsiness, nystagmus, vertigo, and nausea.

Chronic use of this drug may produce the following symptoms: peripheral neuropathy, skin rashes, hyperplasia of the gums, and megaloblastic anemia.

DISOPYRAMIDE PHOSPHATE (NORPACE)[29-31]

Disopyramide has electrophysiological effects similar to those of quinidine but has fewer gastrointestinal side effects. It acts as a direct membrane depressant and as a vagolytic. It is effective in the suppression of PVCs and ventricular tachycardia and less successful in the management of atrial tachyarrhythmias, although it is used successfully to treat paroxysmal supraventricular tachycardia and new onsets of atrial fibrillation (less than 7 days' duration).

Disopyramide prolongs infranodal conduction time (H-Q interval) and atrial and ventricular refractory periods.

Because of its depressant effect on the sinus node, it should be administered cautiously to patients with sinus node dysfunction.

Therapeutic dosage and administration

Disopyramide is eliminated by the kidney and liver with an average half-life of 5 to 6 hours in normal persons. Therapeutic plasma level is 2 to 4 μg/ml. Studies have shown that in patients with myocardial infarction the drug has a reduced clearance and prolonged half-life, probably due to reduced renal function. On this basis, these workers have suggested the following regimen for intravenous administration:

1. First 2 mg/kg over 15 minutes
2. Then 2 mg/kg over the next 45 minutes
3. Next, a maintenance infusion, 0.4 mg/kg/hr
4. Dosage reduced further in patients with greater reductions in creatinine clearance

When taken orally, disopyramide is almost completely absorbed from the gastrointestinal tract, with maximum plasma levels 1 to 3 hours after ingestion. Therapeutic plasma concentrations may be achieved orally with a maintenance dose of 150 mg four times a day. Usually a loading dose is not required. The maximum daily dose should not exceed 1600 mg orally. Dosage should be reduced in patients with impaired renal function.

Side effects

The atropine-like effects of disopyramide are responsible for its most significant side effects, which include a dry mouth and urinary retention.

Contraindications

Disopyramide is contraindicated when there is pulmonary edema, uncontrolled congestive heart failure, cardiogenic shock, glaucoma, and urinary retention. Its effects on the myocardium may be accentuated in hyperkalemic states and it may be harmful to patients with sinus node dysfunction or advanced atrioventricular block.[29]

BRETYLIUM TOSYLATE (BRETYLOL)

Bretylium is a valuable adjunct in the treatment of patients with ventricular fibrillation and ventricular tachycardia who have been resistant to other drugs and electrical countershock.[32]

Bretylium increases the ventricular fibrillatory threshold, action potential duration, and effective refractory period. It restores the resting membrane potential of injured cells toward normal without affecting normal myocardial cells.

Bretylium has a positive inotropic effect on the heart, which sets it apart from other antiarrhythmics.[33]

Therapeutic dosage and administration

Bretylium is excreted unchanged in the urine; consequently the duration of its effect depends partly on renal function.

This drug may be administered intravenously or intramuscularly. Therapeutic effects are achieved at about 5 to 15 mg/kg and may be reduced to 2 or 3 mg/kg after a satisfactory therapeutic response. In some cases even smaller doses are effective.[33]

Toxicity and side effects

When the drug has been administered too rapidly, nausea and vomiting have been reported. The most important side effect is orthostatic hypotension secondary to the action of the drug in blocking postganglionic sympathetic transmission. However, because of the positive inotropic effect of bretylium, there is usually no change in blood pressure as long as the patient is in a reclining position.

DIGITALIS

Digitalis glycosides are of value because of their positive inotropic effect and because of their antiarrhythmic action on the atria and AV junction.

The inotropic effect of digitalis is the result of its depression of sodium-potassium ATPase and the resultant increased influx of calcium into the cell.

The antiarrhythmic action of digitalis is related to its action on intra-atrial and AV conduction and its interaction with the autonomic nervous system.

Digitalis is used to control the ventricular response to atrial fibrillation

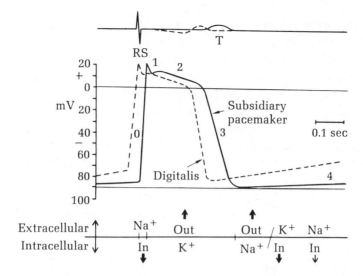

Fig. 18-3. Diagrammatic representation of the effect of digitalis on the action potential and the ECG (broken line). Bottom panel shows the transmembrane cation movement. (From Mason, D., Zelis, R., Lee, G., James, H., Spann, J., and Amsterdam, E.: Am. J. Cardiol. **27:**546, 1971.)

and flutter because it prolongs AV conduction time and AV nodal refractoriness.[34]

Digitalis depresses phase 4 of the action potential in atrial specialized cells and thus may suppress atrial ectopic impulses. It also enhances intra-atrial conduction and thus may abolish intra-atrial reentry.

Digitalis causes sinus slowing because of its antiadrenergic and cholinergic effects. This drug has been shown to decrease the sensitivity of the sinus node to sympathetic stimulation and to enhance vagal excitability.[35]

In the ventricles, digitalis does not have antiarrhythmic effects. On the contrary, it tends to promote ectopic impulse formation by increasing the slope of phase 4 in the cells of the His-Purkinje system.[36] Any remission of ventricular arrhythmias is more than likely secondary to the positive inotropic effect of digitalis.[35]

Effects on the ECG

All the ECG changes are directly related to the changes in the action potential (Fig. 18-3). The primary changes are a sagging of the S-T segment, giving it a scooped appearance, and a shortening of the Q-T interval. S-T segment depression is also seen in myocardial ischemia. However, in this case, the Q-T interval is prolonged.

Therapeutic dosage and administration

The most widely used preparation of digitalis are digoxin and digitoxin.
Digoxin. Digoxin has a half-life of 34 hours and is 75% to 85% absorbed

when given orally. It is excreted unchanged in the urine; thus the factors determining the selection of an appropriate maintenance dose include renal function and lean body mass. Obesity does not require increased dosage, since digoxin is poorly soluble in fat.[37]

Digoxin can accumulate in the body without the administration of a loading dose, and a steady state blood concentration will be reached in 5 to 7 days. The accumulated dose is determined by the maintenance dose. If a loading dose is given, it should be adjusted according to the estimated maintenance dose and be given in divided doses. Generally speaking, the loading dose should be three times the anticipated maintenance dose.

Before changing to digoxin from maintenance with digitoxin, 3 days should elapse between the last dose of digitoxin and the first one of digoxin because the effect of digoxin is superimposed on that of the longer-acting digitoxin, and toxicity may result.[38]

The therapeutic blood level for digoxin is 1 to 2 ng/ml. The potentially toxic blood level is considered to be over 3 ng/ml.[39] Toxicity may, however, occur at therapeutic serum levels after myocardial infarction and in association with hypoxia, hypokalemia, and hypomagnesemia.

Digitoxin. Digitoxin has a half-life of 5 to 7 days. When taken orally, it is 100% absorbed. Its metabolites are excreted in stool and urine.

Therapeutic blood levels for digitoxin are 14 to 30 ng/ml. A potentially toxic blood level is over 30 ng/ml.[39]

Digitalis toxicity

Digitalis at toxic blood levels is thought to bind with sodium-potassium ATPase. This results in a slowing of conduction and acceleration of repolarization secondary to the alteration of potassium gradient across the cell membrane.

Digitalis also causes an increase in the slope of phase 4 in the cells of the specialized conducting system and may thus result in PVCs. Digitalis is also thought to cause the development of delayed afterdepolarizations (p. 29), which may be responsible for the exactly coupled extrasystole,[40] the commonly seen symptom of digitalis toxicity.

Electroshock

Digitalis toxicity. Electroshock in the presence of digitalis toxicity may precipitate ventricular tachycardia or ventricular fibrillation and is contraindicated except as a lifesaving measure.

Digitalized and hypokalemic-hypomagnesemic patients. If the patient is fully digitalized, though not toxic, but is hypokalemic or hypomagnesemic, there is an increased chance of developing ventricular tachycardia or ventricular fibrillation if cardioversion is performed. Therefore cardioversion should be delayed, if at all possible, until these electrolyte abnormalities are corrected.

Digitalized and normal electrolytes. If the patient is fully digitalized and does not have electrolyte abnormalities, cardioversion is not contraindicated. These patients may develop transient PVCs or transient first-degree AV block and should be carefully monitored after cardioversion.

Before elective cardioversion. Before elective cardioversion is performed, digitalis should be withheld for one or two doses (24 hours). If there is some concern that digitalis toxicity may be present, blood levels should be checked. Electrolytes should be checked routinely before cardioversion.

NEW ANTIARRHYTHMIC AGENTS

Table 4 is included to offer a summary of the newest antiarrhythmic agents. Disopyramide is already approved for use in the United States, while the others are candidates.

Electrolytes

With an understanding of the processes involved in maintaining the resting membrane potential in the single cell, one reaches some appreciation of the importance of electrolyte balance in the body. It is through the action of ions on the cell membrane that the depolarization process takes place and electrochemical currents are transmitted within the muscle fibers.

POTASSIUM

Potassium (K^+) is found in abundance in the body. Because of this and because of the ease with which this ion diffuses across the cell membrane, it plays a major role in maintaining the integrity of the cell.

It is excreted by the body in the urine, feces, and perspiration. Therefore diuretics as well as vomiting, diaphoresis, and diarrhea can rapidly deplete the body of this vital ion. An abnormally low potassium content of the blood is called hypokalemia.

Conversely, anuria can cause a potassium buildup, creating an abnormally high potassium concentration (hyperkalemia). Both hyperkalemia and hypokalemia may produce serious arrhythmias and death.

Hyperkalemia

The resting membrane potential is dependent for its strength on the size of the potassium gradient across the membrane. In its resting state there is approximately thirty times as much K^+ within the cell as there is in the extracellular fluid. The action potential is dependent on the strength of the resting membrane potential for its amplitude, or the amount of positive

Table 4. Clinical characteristics of new antiarrhythmic agents*

Drug	Dose — Intravenous	Dose — Oral	Effective serum or plasma concentration (µg/ml)	Elimination half-life (hr)	Absorption	Metabolism secretion route	Side effects	Onset of action — Intravenous (min)	Onset of action — Oral (hr)
Amiodarone	5-10 mg/kg	Maintenance: 200-800 mg	—	—	Fair	—	Ophthalmologic, endocrine, neurologic, dermatologic, cardiovascular	5-10 min	4-6
Aprindine	200 mg at 2 mg/min; 30 min later, 100 mg at 2 mg/min; 6 hr later, 100 mg at 2 mg/min	Loading: 100 mg q 6 hr, day 1; 75 mg q 6 hr, day 2; 50 mg q 6 hr, day 3; Maintenance: 25-50 mg q 8 hr or q 12 hr	1-3	20-30	Good	Hepatic	Neurologic, gastrointestinal, hematologic, cardiovascular	5-10	2
Disopyramide	2 mg/kg	Loading: 300 mg; Maintenance: 150 mg q 6 hr	2-8	5-8	Good	Renal 50%; probably hepatic 50%	Anticholinergic cardiovascular	<5 min	½-3
Ethmozin	Loading: 1-3 mg/kg†	Maintenance: 75-150 mg, q 6 hr‡	0.5-1	5-10	Good†	Probably hepatic†	Neurologic, gastrointestinal, cardiovascular	<5†	2†
Mexiletine	Loading: 1200 mg/12 hr; Maintenance 250-500 mg/12 hr	Loading: 400-600 mg; Maintenance 200-300 mg, q 8 hr	0.5-2.0	10-26	Good	Probably hepatic	Neurologic, gastrointestinal, cardiovascular	<5	1-2
Tocainide	0.5-0.75 mg/kg/min for 15 min	Loading: 400-600 mg; Maintenance: 400-800 mg, q 8 hr	3.5-10	10-17	Good	Renal 40%; probably hepatic 60%	Neurologic, gastrointestinal, cardiovascular	5-10	1½
Verapamil	0.075-0.15 mg/kg	Maintenance: 80-120 mg q 8 hr or q 6 hr	—	3-7	Good	Hepatic	Neurologic, gastrointestinal, cardiovascular	<5	1-2

* From Zipes, D. P., and Troup, P. J.: New antiarrhythmic agents, Am. J. Cardiol. **41:**1006, 1978.
† Animal data.
‡ According to studies in progress, maintenance doses may be in the range of 250 mg every 8 hours and provide a slightly longer half-life.

overshoot, and for the rate of rise of this amplitude. Conduction velocity is in turn dependent on rapid depolarization. Neighborning fibers are stimulated faster by a strong action potential with a steep rise (phase 0).

In summary, the resting membrane potential, action potential, and conduction velocity are all dependent for their strength and speed on the potassium gradient.

Hyperkalemia (elevated levels of extracellular K^+) causes the gradient of that ion across the cell membrane to be lessened. This causes the resting membrane potential to be lowered, and this in turn reduces phase 0 of the action potential and slows conduction. The characteristic effect of hyperkalemia is therefore slow conduction (intra-atrial, atrioventricular, and/or intraventricular heart block).

Furthermore, the velocity of phase 3 is increased and the action potential

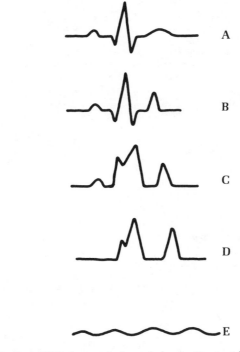

Fig. 18-4. ECG changes in hyperkalemia. See text for explanation.

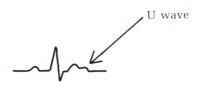

Fig. 18-5. *U wave* seen in hypokalemia.

duration shortened, both of which are considered to be the cause of the characteristic narrowing and peaking of the T wave when the serum potassium exceeds 5.5 mEq/L.

Potassium is also known to have antiarrhythmic properties. Mild hyperkalemia (6.0 to 6.5 mEq/L) enhances AV conduction and thus may interrupt a reentry pathway or improve AV conduction in patients with heart block.

ECG changes

1. The normal serum K⁺ is 4 to 5.5 mEq/L (Fig. 18-4, *A*).
2. Changes start early (K⁺ 6 mEq/L), with a peaked T wave and a normal QRS complex and P-R interval (Fig. 18-4, *B*).
3. The QRS widens and is slurred (K⁺ 7 to 7.5 mEq/L) (Fig. 18-4, *C*).
4. Atrial conduction ceases and the P wave is not seen. The broad QRS persists (K⁺ 8 mEq/L) (Fig. 18-4, *D*).
5. The sine (curved) wave is seen as a terminal event (Fig. 18-4, *E*).

Table 5. Effect of drugs and electrolytes on the ECG*

Drug or electrolyte	QRS complex	S-T segment	P wave	T wave	U wave	P-R segment	Q-T interval
Digitalis		Sagging		Flattens		Prolongs	Shortens
Quinidine	Widens (toxic)	Depresses	Widens and notches (toxic)	Flattens or inverts			Prolongs
Propranolol				Normal or slightly higher		Prolongs	Shortens
Phenytoin						Shortens	Shortens
Disopyramide	Widens		Widens			Prolongs	
Potassium							
Hyperkalemia	Widens	Depresses (>6.5 mEq/L)	Widens (>7.5 mEq/L)	Tall and peaked (5.5-6.5 mEq/L)		Prolongs (>7.5 mEq/L)	
Hypokalemia		Sagging		Notching, then inversion	Prominent		Prolongs (due to U wave)
Calcium							
Hypercalcemia				Widens and rounds			Shortens
Hypocalcemia							Prolongs
Magnesium	Widens (toxic)			Flattens		Prolongs (toxic)	
Lithium				Flattens			

*From Tilkian, S. M., Conover, M. B., and Tilkian, A. G.: Laboratory tests, ed. 2, St. Louis, 1979, The C. V. Mosby Co.

Hypokalemia

The effects of hypokalemia are mainly the result of loss of the potassium gradient across the cell membrane and the effect of this loss on the action potential. Automaticity is increased, and there is an interference with the normal repolarization process, causing ectopic beats and changes in the S-T segment and T wave.

There is a prominent *U wave* (a positive deflection immediately following or at the end of the T wave). The Q-T interval often appears prolonged because of the superimposition of the U wave on the T. The true Q-T interval is of normal duration in hypokalemia (Fig. 18-5).

CALCIUM

The level of myocardial contractility is thought to be determined by the number of calcium ions available. There are four proteins involved in the process of myocardial contraction: myosin, actin, tropomyosin, and troponin. Contraction is inhibited by the combination of troponin-tropomyosin. The contractile process is initiated when calcium released by excitation of the cell membrane becomes bound to troponin. Therefore calcium has a direct effect on myocardial contractility. Increased extracellular calcium improves cardiac contractility. In levels exceeding the body's tolerance, it would produce rigor of the myocardium.

ECG changes due to hypercalcemia are so slight as to be of no diagnostic value. In hypocalcemia, repolarization is prolonged, causing a duration of the Q-T interval that is beyond normal limits.

MAGNESIUM

Hypomagnesemia usually accompanies hypokalemia. Hypermagnesemia may cause flattening of the T wave and, in very toxic levels, PR and QRS widening. Table 5 summarizes the effect of drugs and electrolytes on the ECG.

References

ALPHA AND BETA ADRENERGIC RECEPTORS

1. Ahlquist, R. P.: A study of the adrenotropic receptors, Am. J. Physiol. **153**:586, 1948.
2. Lands, A. M., Arnold, A., Meauliff, J. P., Ludeuna, F. P., and Brown, R. G., Jr: Differentiation of receptor systems activated by sympathomimetic amines, Nature **214**:597, 1967.
3. Ahlquist, R. P.: Present state of alpha- and beta-adrenergic drugs. I. The adrenergic receptors. In Appraisal and Reappraisal of Cardiac Therapy Series, edited by DeGraff,

A. C., and Frieden, J.: Am. Heart J. **92**:661, 1976.
4. Wit, A. L., Hoffman, B. F., and Rosen, M. R.: Electrophysiology and pharmacology of cardiac arrhythmias. IX. Cardiac electrophysiologic effects of beta-adrenergic receptor stimulation and blockade, Part A. In Appraisal and Reappraisal of Cardiac Therapy, edited by DeGraff, A. C., and Frieden, J.: Am. Heart J. **90**:521, 1975.
5. Prichard, B. N. C.: Beta adrenergic receptor blocking drugs in angina pectoris, Drugs **7**: 55, 1974.

6. Sonnenblick, E. H., Frishman, W. H., and LeJemtel, T. H.: Dobutamine: a new synthetic cardioactive sympathetic amine, Med. Intell. **300:**17, 1979.

7. Ahlquist, R. P.: Present state of alpha- and beta-adrenergic drugs. II. The adrenergic blocking agents. In Appraisal and Reappraisal of Cardiac Therapy Series, edited by DeGraff, A. C., and Frieden, J.: Am. Heart J. **92:**804, 1976.

8. Ahlquist, R. P.: Present state of alpha- and beta-adrenergic drugs. III. Beta blocking agents. In Appraisal and Reappraisal of Cardiac Therapy Series, edited by DeGraff, A. C., and Frieden, J.: Am. Heart J. **93:**117, 1977.

9. Wit, A. L., Hoffman, B. R., and Rosen, M. R.: Electrophysiology and pharmacology of cardiac arrhythmias. IX. Cardiac electrophysiologic effects of beta-adrenergic receptor stimulation and blockade, Part B. In Appraisal and Reappraisal of Cardiac Therapy Series, edited by DeGraff, A. C., and Frieden, J.: Am. Heart J. **90:**665, 1975.

10. Hjalmarson, A., and Waagstein, F.: The advantage of beta$_1$ stimulation (prenalterol) and beta$_1$ blockade (metoprolol) in the treatment of patients with ischemic heart disease (abstr.), Am. J. Cardiol. **43:**415, 1979.

11. Canepa-Anson, R., Bourdillon, P. D., and Rickards, A. F.: Hemodynamic effects of intravenous metoprolol (abstr.), Am. J. Cardiol. **43:**381, 1979.

LIDOCAINE

12. Southworth, J. L., McKusick, V. A., Peirce, E. C., and Rawson, F. L., Jr.: Ventricular fibrillation precipitated by cardiac catheterization, J.A.M.A. **143:**717, 1950.

13. Kupersmith, J., Parodi, E., and Hoffman, B. F.: In vivo electrophysiologic effects of lidocaine in canine acute myocardial infarction, Circ. Res. **36:**84, 1975.

14. El-Sherif, N., Scherlag, B. J., Lazzara, R., and Hope, R. R.: Re-entrant ventricular arrhythmias in the late myocardial infarction period. 4. Mechanism of action of lidocaine, Circulation **56:**395, 1977.

15. Rosen, M. R., Hoffman, B. F., and Wit, A. L.: Electrophysiology and pharmacology of cardiac arrhythmias. V. Cardiac antiarrhythmic effects of lidocaine, Am. Heart J. **89:**526, 1975.

16. Wyman, M. G., et al.: Multiple bolus technique for lidocaine administration during the first hours of an acute myocardial infarction, Am. J. Cardiol. **41:**313, 1978.

17. Harrison, D. C.: Should lidocaine be administered routinely to all patients after acute myocardial infarction? Circulation **58:**583, 1978.

18. Woosley, R. L., and Shand, D. G.: Pharmacokinetics of antiarrhythmic drugs, Am. J. Cardiol. **41:**986, 1978.

19. Wyman, M. G., and Hammersmith, L.: Comprehensive treatment plan for the prevention of primary ventricular fibrillation in acute myocardial infarction, Am. J. Cardiol. **33:**661, 1974,

20. Wyman, M. G.: Lidocaine, Circulation. (in press.)

PROCAINAMIDE AND QUINIDINE

21. Ueda, C. T., Hirschfeld, D. S., Scheinman, M. M., et al.: Disposition kinetics of quinidine, Clin. Pharmacol. Ther. **19:**30, 1976.

22. Hordof, A. J., Edie, R., Malm, J. R., Hoffman, B. F., and Rosen, M. R.: Electrophysiologic properties and response to pharmacologic agents of fibers from diseased human atria, Circulation **54:**775, 1976.

23. Wu, D., Denes, P., Bauernfeind, R., K., Amat-y-Leon, F., and Rosen, K. M.: Effects of procainamide on atrioventricular nodal re-entrant paroxysmal tachycardia, Circulation **57:**1171, 1978.

24. Hoffman, B. F., Rosen, M. R., and Wit, A. L.: Electrophysiology and pharmacology of cardiac arrhythmias. VII. Cardiac effects of quinidine and procainamide, Part A. and B, Am. Heart J. **89:**804; **90:**117, 1975.

25. Greenblatt, D. J., Pfeifer, H. J., Ochs, H. R., et al.: Pharmacokinetics of quinidine in humans after intravenous, intramuscular and oral administration, J. Pharma. Exp. Ther. **202:**365, 1977.

26. Data, J. L., Wilkinson, G. R., and Nies, A. S.: Interaction of quinidine with anticonvulsive drugs, N. Engl. J. Med. **294:**699, 1976.

27. El-Sherif, N., and Lazzara, R.: Re-entrant ventricular arrhythmias in the late myocardial infarction period 5. Mechanism of action of dephenylhydantoin, Circulation **57:**465, 1978.

28. Wit, A. L., Rosen, M. R., and Hoffman, B. F.: Electrophysiology and pharmacology of cardiac arrhythmias. VIII. Cardiac effects of diphenylhydantoin, Parts A and B. Am. Heart J. **90:**265, 397, 1975.

DISOPYRAMIDE

29. Yu, P. N.: Disopyramide phosphate (Norpace): a new antiarrhythmic drug, Circulation **59:**236, 1979.
30. Ward, J. W., and Kinghom, C. R.: The pharmacokinetics of disopyramide following myocardial infarction, with special reference to oral and intravenous dose regimens, J. Int. Med. Res. **4**(supp. 1):49, 1976.
31. Rangno, R. E., Wamich, W., Ogolvoe, R.: et al.: Correlation of disopyramide pharmacokinetics with efficacy in ventricular tachyarrhythmias, J. Int. Med. Res. 4(Supp. 1):54, 1976.

BRETYLIUM

32. Holder, D. A., Sniderman, A. D., Fraser, G., and Fällen, E. L.: Experience with bretylium tosylate by a hospital cardiac arrest team, Circulation **55:**541, 1977.
33. Baganer, M. B.: Treatment of ventricular fibrillation and other acute arrhythmias with bretylium tosylate, Am. J. Cardiol. **21:**530, 1968.

DIGITALIS

34. Hoffman, B. F.: Effects of digitalis on electrical activity of cardiac membranes. In Marks, B. H., and Weissler, A. M., editors: Basic and clinical pharmacology of digitalis, Springfield, Ill., 1972, Charles C Thomas, Publisher.
35. Rosen, M. R., Wit, A. L., and Hoffman, B. F.: Electrophysiology and pharmacology of cardiac arrhythmias. IV. Cardiac antiarrthythmic and toxic effects of digitalis, Am. Heart J. **89:**391, 1975.
36. Vassalle, M., Karis, J., and Hoffman, B. F.: Toxic effects of ouabain on Purkinje fibers and ventricular muscle fibers, Am. J. Physiol. **203:**433, 1962.
37. Marcus, F. I.: Current concepts of digoxin therapy, Mod. Concepts Cardiovasc. Dis. **45** (2):77, 1976.
38. Marcus, F. I.: Digitalis pharmacokinetics and metabolism, Am. J. Med. **58:**452, 1975.
39. Tilkian, S. M., Conover, M. H., and Tilkian, A. G.: Clinical implications of laboratory tests, ed. 2, 1979, The C. V. Mosby Co.
40. Cranefield, P. F.: Action potentials, afterpotentials, and arrhythmias, Circ. Res. **41:**415, 1977.

CHAPTER 19

Accidental electrocution

The exact number of fatal and nonfatal electrical accidents involving cardiac monitoring equipment will never be known. This is not only due to the natural inclination to underreport such incidents, but also, more importantly, to the fact that personnel can be involved in, and actually cause, an accident without being aware of their implication in the incident.

As more monitoring equipment is brought into use, it becomes imperative that greater effort be made to minimize the possibility of electrical shock to the patient.

The electrically sensitive patient

The primary reason for the increased shock hazard in the critical care areas is the use of transvenous intracardiac catheters that provide a direct electrical connection to the myocardium. Such a direct connection of the heart to the outside environment creates what is referred to as the *electrically sensitive patient*. Because the cardiac tissue is directly exposed, the patient is rendered extremely vulnerable to a level of electrical shock that is imperceptible to a person without a cardiac catheter.

In order to fully appreciate the susceptibility of the electrically sensitive patient and the precautions necessary to protect this patient, an understanding of the nature of electrical current flow and the potential hazards is necessary.

Electrical current flow

Current flow is the movement of electrons around a closed loop that consists of a two-terminal voltage source and a conductive path connecting these terminals. Conductive paths are formed by metallic and/or ionic conductors and exhibit resistance to the flow of current. Following is an outline of some conductors that would be encountered in the cardiac care unit (CCU) or intensive care unit (ICU).

TYPICAL CONDUCTORS FOUND IN THE CCU/ICU

1. Ionic conductors
   a. Saline

   b. Urine
   c. Blood
   d. Metal furniture, beds, lights, and instruments
2. Metallic conductors
   a. Pacing catheters
   b. ECG needle electrodes
   c. Catheter metal guide wires
   d. Metal furniture, beds, lights and instruments

OHM'S LAW

The relationship between the applied voltage, path resistance, and resultant current flow is known as Ohm's law. Mathematically the relationship is represented by the following equation:

$$\text{Current (I)} = \frac{\text{Voltage (V)}}{\text{Resistance (R)}}$$

Briefly, this expression states that the current flow increases as the applied voltage is increased and decreases as the circuit path resistance is increased. The units of measurement involved are volts (V), the unit of voltage; ohms, the unit of resistance; and amperes (A), the unit of current. The usual scaling prefixes such as milli- (1/1000), micro- (1/1,000,000), kilo- (1000), and mega- (1,000,000) are used with these units. Just as a milligram is one thousandth of a gram, a milliampere (mA) is one thousandth of an ampere. The prefixes kilo- and mega-, for the purposes of this discussion, apply only to resistance. The examples in Fig. 19-1 illustrate the effect of changing resistance and voltage on current flow.

Wiring systems

The power used for operating electrical equipment within the hospital is 120-V, 60-Hz alternating current. This power is available at the standard three-pin wall receptacle and is connected to the equipment by the usual three-pronged plug and line cord (Fig. 19-2).

The longer round pin is the grounding or ground pin and plays an important part in patient safety. One of the flat blades is the *hot* connecting pin, and the other is the *neutral* connecting pin. In the two-wire system this ground pin is absent, causing serious electrical hazards, which will be discussed later.

Alternating current (AC) flow. The hot connecting pin is constantly changing from positive to negative and back again, while the neutral is changing from negative to positive and back. The two are always out of step (one is positive at the same time that the other is negative); therefore the

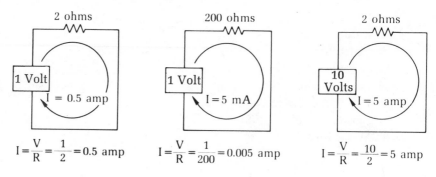

$$I = \frac{V}{R} = \frac{1}{2} = 0.5 \text{ amp} \qquad I = \frac{V}{R} = \frac{1}{200} = 0.005 \text{ amp} \qquad I = \frac{V}{R} = \frac{10}{2} = 5 \text{ amp}$$

Fig. 19-1. Effect of changing resistance and voltage on current flow.

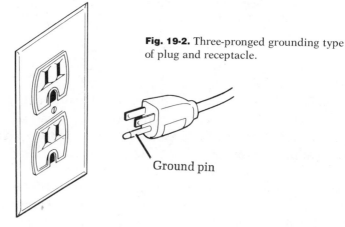

Fig. 19-2. Three-pronged grounding type of plug and receptacle.

Ground pin

resultant current flow is constantly changing, or *alternating*, in direction and hence the term *alternating current*. Sixty of these alternating cycles take place in a second—thus the designation 60 Hz.

In discussing AC current flow, these alternations are ignored, and the current is simply considered to be flowing from the hot connection through one conductor of the line cord to the equipment, then returning through another conductor of the line cord to the neutral connection. Note that in this example no current flows through the ground connection.

Ground

The earth itself is a conductor of electricity, albeit a poor one. Its conductivity is caused by the moisture and resultant ions in the soil and by an extensive network of conductive metal water pipes, gas pipes, conduits, and so on. It is this network that is referred to as *ground*.

If only for safety reasons, it is obvious that the electrical power distribution system must take this conductive ground network into consideration.

Table 6. Effect of shock current on the heart

Current	Through intact skin (macroshock)	Direct contact to myocardium (microshock)
10 A	⎫ Sustained myocardial contraction	
5 A	⎭	
2 A	⎫	
1 A	⎪	
500 mA	⎬ Ventricular fibrillation (respiration continues)	
200 mA	⎪	
100 mA	⎭	
50 mA	——— Pain, fainting, exhaustion	
20 mA	——— *Let go* current (muscle contraction)	
10 mA		
5 mA	Maximum harmless current	⎫ Ventricular fibrillation (humans)
2 mA		⎭ (2.5 cm. diam. plate electrode)
1 mA	——— Threshold of perception	Ventricular fibrillation (humans)
500 μA		⎫ (0.25 cm. diam. plate electrode)
200 μA		⎭ Ventricular fibrillation in dogs
100 μA		⎫ (catheter)
50 μA		⎪
20 μA		⎭
10 μA	————————————————	Maximum current recommended
5 μA		for electrically safe areas*

*Association for Advancement of Medical Instrumentation (AAMI), type A.

The method used is one that results in the neutral wire being connected to ground or grounded at the power distribution transformer. While this approach provides a safe solution for the large majority of power users, it does present a degree of hazard: any grounded item is a potential circuit path.

Electrical shock

The operation of the heart is dependent on internally generated electrical pulses. The effect of electrical shock is to repetitively stimulate the heart during the vulnerable T wave and cause ventricular fibrillation. In cases of very severe shock the heart is completely stopped by sustained contraction. The severity of an electrical shock is related to the current density through the tissue involved. The shock can vary from an intensity that is almost imperceptible (low current density) to one that is fatal (high current density). Various studies have been made on the effect of electrical shock on both humans and dogs, and the results of some of these studies are summarized in Table 6.

MACROSHOCK

Gross electrical shock is the type in which the current passes through the trunk, with contact to the source being made through intact skin. In this situation the current spreads throughout all of the tissue in its path, and the amount of current that flows through cardiac tissue is a very small fraction of the total. The intact skin exhibits a resistance to the current that ranges from 1000 ohms (for conditions of good contact and moist skin) to 1 million ohms (1 megohm) (for dry skin and low relative humidity).

Body defenses against macroshock. The body has two defenses against electrical shock. First, the high resistance of the skin reduces the amount of current that can flow as the result of a given impressed voltage (Ohm's law). Therefore contact with even full 120-V line voltage generally results in a painful but nonfatal shock. Second, there is a spreading effect whereby the current is distributed throughout the tissue in its path, reducing the current density. Because of this spreading, the cardiac tissue is exposed to only a small fraction of the current passing through the body.

Taking these protective mechanisms into account, electrical safety standards have been established and implemented. The success of these standards is demonstrated by the fact that despite the extensive use of electrical equipment, serious shock due to normal use of modern equipment in good repair is very rare. However effective these standards have been for the protection of the uncatheterized person, they are not adequate to ensure the safety of the electrically sensitive patient. To protect these patients, an electrically safe area must be created for them in which more stringent standards are maintained.

MICROSHOCK

The electrically sensitive patient is susceptible to current levels that are imperceptible to the normal person. Studies have shown that ventricular fibrillation can be induced in a catheterized patient with current levels below 1 mA (Table 6). This greatly increased vulnerability of the electrically sensitive patient to electrical shock results from broaching the body's two defenses—skin resistance and the spreading effect of current. First, the use of a catheter can reduce the path resistance from the normal 1000-ohm to 1-megohm range to a 500- to 1000-ohm range. Second, and more critical, instead of the current spreading through the body and thus diminishing, all current is concentrated in the heart at the point of catheter contact, resulting in high current density.

Due to extremely small currents involved in the microshock environment, a potentially lethal condition can exist and not be perceived by uncatheterized persons coming into contact with the current source or becoming part of the current path. As can be seen in Table 6, the imperceptible current of 1 mA can cause fibrillation. It is this inability of operating personnel to determine when a dangerous condition exists that makes a periodic inspection program and special procedures necessary to ensure patient safety.

Sources of currents

After discussion of the nature of AC microcurrent flow and its effect on the electrically sensitive patient, a question arises as to the origin of these currents. Once the sources of these dangerous currents are known, steps may be taken to locate and eliminate them.

LEAKAGE CURRENTS

Capacitive leakage. The most probable source of currents dangerous to the electrically sensitive patient is what are generally referred to as leakage currents. Although the term suggests that some kind of malfunction must exist in a piece of electrical equipment in order for it to "leak" current, the leakage is in fact the result of a normal electrical characteristic known as capacitive coupling—the characteristic of coupling AC current through an insulator. Whenever an AC voltage is impressed between two electrical conductors that are in close proximity, a current flows through the conductors, even though they are perfectly insulated from each other. The amount of current flow depends on several parameters. Among these are the amount of separation between the conductors (the less the separation, the greater the current flow), the effective area of the conductors (the greater the common area, the greater the current flow), and the impressed voltage (the greater the impressed voltage, the greater the current flow).

Most equipment has leakage current to its metal case or to any metallic items on a plastic case unless it has been specially designed to eliminate this hazard. For the types and sizes of equipment in use in the unit, these capacitive leakage currents are small and harmless to operating personnel and patients who are not electrically sensitive. However, the electrically sensitive patient is susceptible to harm at these current levels.

Resistive leakage. The amount of leakage current increases when the equipment is subjected to a humid environment, moisture, dust, or a corrosive atmosphere. These cause the deterioration of insulation used in the equipment and consequently lower the insulation resistance. This type of leakage is known as resistance leakage. It is different from, but can occur in addition to, the capacitive leakage discussed earlier. The result is that the two leakages add and increase the shock hazard, at times to the point at which the equipment is hazardous even to the person who is not electrically sensitive. Equipment that is subject to adverse environmental conditions, such as vacuum cleaners, floor waxers, and pumps, can develop high leakage currents.

Protection from leakage currents. In order to protect the user from such leakage currents, the metallic case of the equipment is connected by a separate wire in the line cord to the ground pin of the outlet. Leakage current is then conducted harmlessly to ground. This protection is available only in a three-wire system. Two-wire systems have no path to dissipate leakage currents and constitute a safety hazard.

EQUIPMENT FAULTS

Faults (shorts) are actual malfunctions of the equipment, whereby an internal conductor comes in contact with another conductor or with the case. The situation that causes a shock hazard is a fault to the case or housing. Depending on the point in the circuit at which the fault occurs, the voltage on the case can range from 120 V to a few millivolts.

The method of protection here is the same as for leakage currents, that is, grounding the case with a three-pin power plug. The fault current is then conducted harmlessly to ground. It is obvious that if the fault current were large, the circuit breaker or fuse supplying the current would open, interrupting the current and publicizing the malfunction. What is not obvious is that substantial current can flow without opening the circuit breaker or fuse because circuit breakers or fuses are designed to carry 15 to 20 A without opening. Unless the total of normal current and fault current exceeds this rating, no opening will occur. In many instances the faulty equipment will continue to operate normally or give a slightly degraded performance. However, if the grounding circuit should ever be broken, a hazard is present for the electrically sensitive patient that could also affect the operating personnel.

This ground connection is the mainstay of patient safety. However, it is effective only to the extent that it provides an extremely low resistance path to a true ground. Hence it is necessary that a well-designed grounding system be used and maintained in the areas where patients are susceptible to microshock.

Typical hazardous situations

After investigating the sources of potentially dangerous currents and determining the levels of current that can be a threat to the electrically sensitive patient, it is helpful to explore potentially dangerous situations that may arise in the CCU.

UNGROUNDED EQUIPMENT

Ungrounded equipment can be readily identified by its use of a two-pronged rather than a three-pronged plug. The two-pronged plug has no provision for routing any leakage or fault current safely to the power grounding system. If a piece of ungrounded equipment is defective, it can pose a hazard to the nonelectrically sensitive patient and to the operating personnel, as well as to the electrically sensitive patient. When it is functioning

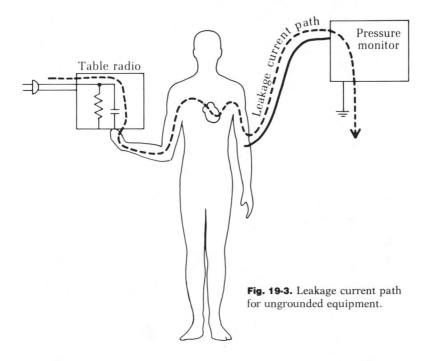

Table radio

Leakage current path

Pressure
monitor

Fig. 19-3. Leakage current path
for ungrounded equipment.

normally and is in good repair, ungrounded equipment is still a hazard to
the electrically sensitive patient. For example, consider the patient who has
a pacemaker or an indwelling catheter for cardiac pressure monitoring. The
catheter, through its associated monitor, provides a resistance to ground
that is sufficiently low to allow the *leakage current* of an ungrounded *table
radio* to pass through the heart if contact is made with the conductive case
of the radio (Fig. 19-3).

EQUIPMENT WITH A DEFECTIVE GROUND

The hazards posed by equipment with open or defective grounding systems are similar to those posed by ungrounded equipment. Although ungrounded equipment can be readily identified and removed, the identification of equipment with an open ground is not as easy. A visual inspection of
power cords is helpful, but to ensure patient safety, a resistance measurement must be made of all grounds.

As in the previous case of a grounded pressure catheter, a defective
ground on an electric bed would allow a dangerous current to flow through
the patient's heart if an attendant were to touch the bare pacemaker terminal while holding the bed rail (Fig. 19-4). It should be noted that some authorities question the use of electric beds in an electrically safe area. It is
thought that the hazard outweighs the convenience.

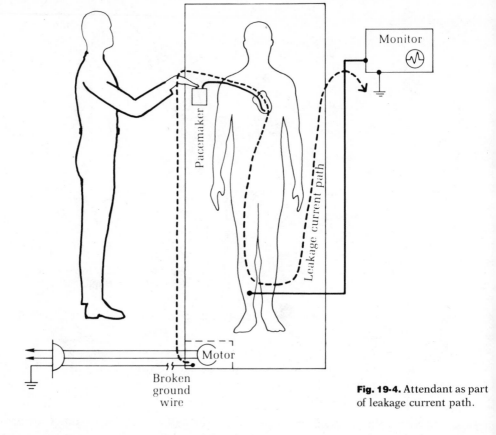

Fig. 19-4. Attendant as part of leakage current path.

UNEQUAL GROUND POTENTIALS

Throughout most of the previous discussion one ground was considered to be the same as any other, at least within the cardiac care unit. To ensure patient safety, it is necessary that the various grounds associated with a given patient be at, or at least very close to, the same electrical potential. Failure to meet this requirement will allow a current to pass through the patient who is connected to two pieces of equipment that are connected to two different grounds. For example, if a patient were connected to a pressure monitor transducer that is normally grounded and to an electrocardiograph machine that has the usual right-leg ground, a current due to the difference in ground potentials could flow through his heart (Fig. 19-5).

The detection of potential differences between receptacle grounds is made more difficult because the potential is usually associated with a high leakage current flowing through the ground system. This leakage current may come from equipment that is not in the unit. In addition, the equipment causing the leakage current may not be in continuous operation, with the result that the difference in ground potentials varies.

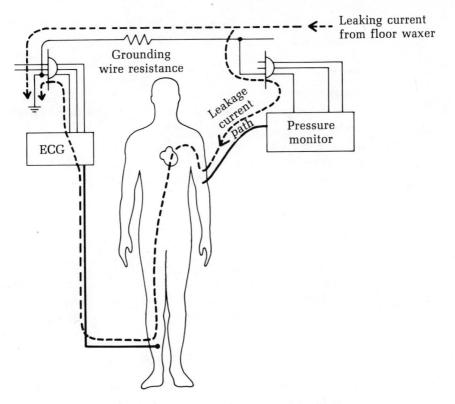

Fig. 19-5. Current flow due to unequal ground potentials.

What can be done to avoid accidental electrocution

Paramount to achieving a safe environment for the electrically sensitive patient is the establishment of an electrically safe area. Within this area special precautions should be enforced with regard to nursing techniques, plant wiring, equipment selection, inspection and maintenance procedures, and training of personnel.

NURSING TECHNIQUE

Do not become part of a circuit that could allow current to flow through you and then through the patient. The following considerations will help to avoid such a potentially fatal situation:

1. Be aware that pressure catheters, intracardiac electrodes, and pacing catheters provide a direct electrical connection to the patient's heart.
2. Insulate all metal terminals, guide wires, and uninsulated electrode wires as follows:
   a. Place plastic or rubber sleeving over exposed terminals.

b. Wear surgical gloves whenever it is necessary to handle bare electrode wires or terminals.

c. Place external battery-powered pacemakers in a surgical glove or plastic sheet to insulate their terminals.

3. When taking an intracardiac ECG, be certain that the intracardiac is connected to the V lead and not to the indifferent (right-leg) electrode.

4. Be aware that intraesophageal and intratracheal devices, due to their close proximity to the posterior myocardium, present a hazard almost as great as that of intracardiac catheters and should be treated with the same care.

5. Maintain a continuing survey of the condition of equipment within the unit.

a. If a tingling sensation (mild electrical shock) is felt when a piece of equipment is touched, it is an indication that the equipment is defective and poses a definite shock hazard to the patient. If not required for life support, the equipment should be removed from the area and tagged to alert others to the danger. When it is required for life support, it should be preferably replaced or repaired as soon as possible.

b. The condition of all power cords and plugs should be noted. The hospital electrician should repair or replace all frayed or damaged cords. Any equipment using two-pronged plugs should be removed *from the hospital* until the plugs can be replaced with the three-pronged grounding type.

6. Do not allow patient-supplied appliances in the unit unless they are battery-powered and not connected to the AC power.

7. Do not run heavy-wheeled equipment over power cords, thus damaging them.

8. Do not store equipment in a manner that exposes the power cords to kinking or extremes of temperature.

9. Avoid the use of extension cords if at all possible.

a. Two-wire extension cords defeat the grounding scheme of the equipment.

b. A three-wire cord *with an open ground* actually generates a leakage current and places it on the case of an otherwise safe piece of equipment.

c. If use of an extension cord is absolutely necessary, it must be the three-wire type and inspected often for an intact grounding wire.

10. Appearance of AC interference on the ECG tracing can result from several causes. Some of these pose a hazard to the patient; others do not. In either event, the interference makes the tracing difficult to

interpret, and the situation should be corrected at once. In an electrically safe area the usual cause of AC interference is dried out electrode pads or a defective patient cable. If not, it may be caused by poorly grounded or defective electrical equipment in use on the patient. By systematically disconnecting and then reconnecting each piece of equipment until the interference disappears, the offending piece of equipment can be identified. Since the presence of AC interference can indicate a shock hazard, equipment causing such interference should be removed from the unit and repaired.

PLANT WIRING

In the electrically safe area all receptacles must be of the three-pin grounding type. The technique of using the wiring conduit or a small-gauge wire for grounding purposes is inadequate for this area. A separate 12-gauge wire should be used for ground. To equalize the grounds at a given bed at the same potential, all the ground wires from outlets serving that bed should be grounded at a single point, and that ground should not connect to outlets other than those serving that bed. All exposed metal items such as water

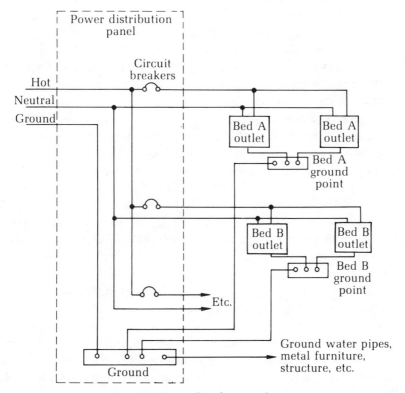

Fig. 19-6. Power distribution scheme.

pipes, building structure, and metal furniture must be connected to a room ground (Fig. 19-6).

Isolation transformers have been proposed for some applications and do have certain advantages. However, the isolation is degraded by both the using equipment and the power distribution wiring, and the transformers themselves are not entirely free of leakage. In order to ensure that equipment failure has not compromised the isolation, monitors must be installed.

Ground fault interrupters of the type used in commercial and industrial buildings do not have adequate sensitivity to protect the electrically sensitive patient. Additionally, automatic power interruption of life support equipment may be a greater hazard than that of shock.

The use of high-sensitivity ground current monitors especially designed for CCU/ICU application provides a continuous check of equipment leakage on the circuit, thus allowing defective equipment to be identified as dangerous before an accident occurs.

EQUIPMENT SELECTION

Equipment used for ECG monitoring has continually improved with respect to features that enhance both diagnostic usefulness and patient safety. Early ECG monitors that used a grounded input posed a hazard if the potential between the electrically sensitive patient and the monitor exceeded 10 mV. Later development of the driven right-leg circuits provided patient protection for voltages up to 500 mV. Since typical voltages that result in differences in ground potentials seldom exceed 1 V, a measure of protection from this hazard is afforded the patient.

The ECG monitor with isolated input circuitry has input amplifiers that are greatly isolated from the rest of the monitor. This is accomplished by means of special circuitry that supplies operating power to the input amplifier and couples the signal to the display on the scope. As a result, the patient is protected against hazardous currents even though the potential between the patient and monitor is full-line voltage (120 V). The patient would thus be protected in the case of a broken grounding wire. Similarly, the hazard posed by a grounded pressure catheter and associated monitor (Fig. 19-3) can be reduced substantially by the use of an isolated pressure monitor.

Telemetry techniques are used in some ECG monitors. In this type of equipment the input amplifier and a telemetry transmitter are combined in a small unit that is worn by the patient. The entire patient unit is powered by a battery, so that complete isolation from the power lines and their attendant hazards is provided. The patient unit sends out a radio signal that is received by the monitor and displayed. Such a system allows the patient to be ambulatory.

The responsibility for a final decision as to the selection of new equipment and other capital improvements usually rests with hospital administrators whose primary field of expertise is, in a broad sense, business management. In order to make rational decisions regarding equipment, administrators must either gain expertise in this technical field or seek outside counsel. The latter course is usually the most efficient. Needless to say, the consultant should be both technically competent and unbiased and be made aware of the hospital's insistence on a safe environment for the electrically sensitive patient.

PERSONNEL TRAINING

While it is certainly true that proper wiring and equipment play an important part in determining patient safety in the electrically safe area, all personnel working within this area must be made aware of (1) the acute vulnerability of the electrically sensitive patient and (2) the part they themselves play in maintaining a safe environment for their patient. Particular emphasis should be placed on nursing technique and on the continuing in-unit inspection of equipment.

INSPECTION

To maintain a continuing high level of patient safety, it is necessary to initiate a system of periodic inspections. These inspections must cover both the electrically safe area and any equipment that may be brought into it. The main object of the inspection is to ensure that none of the equipment can subject the patient to a current of greater than 10 microamperes (μA), As shown in Table 6, the accepted maximum safe current level for an electrically sensitive patient has been established at 10 μA.

The amount of current a patient could receive can be determined by measuring the voltage across a 500-ohm resistor (an amount that simulates the resistance of the patient) connected between the case of an instrument and true ground. This measurement is repeated for all metal surfaces and terminals in the electrically safe area. Ohm's law is used to determine the maximum allowable voltage corresponding to a current of 10 μA and a resistance of 500 ohms. When these parameters are substituted in the equation $V = I \times R$, a value of 5 mV is obtained. Additional measurements should be made to ensure that all receptacle grounds are within 5 mV of each other. Although the measurements described are relatively straightforward, special equipment, fixtures, and techniques are required. Unless the hospital is large enough to maintain this equipment and expertise, outside professional assistance should be engaged.

CHAPTER 20

Test tracings

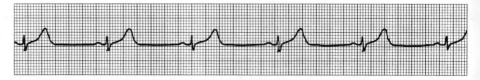

Fig. 1. SINUS BRADYCARDIA. The rate is 48. Rhythm is regular and conduction is normal.

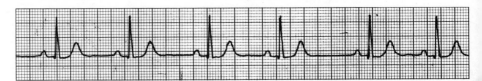

Fig. 2. SINUS ARRHYTHMIA. The rhythm is irregular. The P-P interval at the beginning of the tracing is a full large square (0.20 sec) shorter than the P-P interval at the end of the tracing. The rate is approximately 60 beats/min. Conduction is normal.

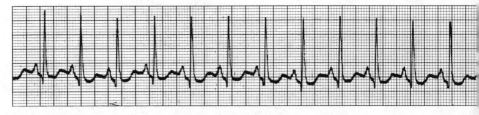

Fig. 3. SINUS TACHYCARDIA. The rate of the sinus node is 110. Conduction is normal.

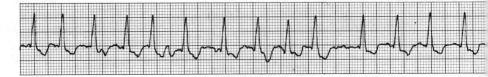

Fig. 4. ATRIAL FIBRILLATION. The absence of P waves and the presence of an irregular ventricular response make a diagnosis of atrial fibrillation certain.

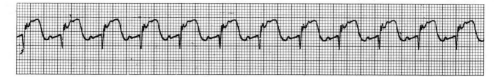

Fig. 5. ATRIAL TACHYCARDIA WITH 2:1 AV CONDUCTION. The atrial rate is 200. There are two P' waves for every QRS complex, and a ventricular rate of 100. One P' wave is apparent just before the QRS complex. The other is on the S-T segment.

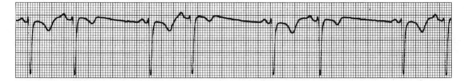

Fig. 6. BIGEMINAL PACS. Every other P wave is premature.

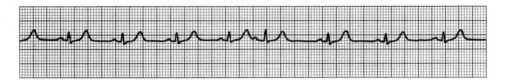

Fig. 7. PAC. The single P' wave in this tracing immediately follows a T wave.

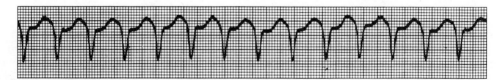

Fig. 8. VENTRICULAR TACHYCARDIA. The tracing consists of a continuous series of ventricular ectopic beats at a rate of 120.

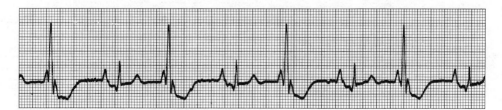

Fig. 9. VENTRICULAR BIGEMINY. These bigeminal ventricular extrasystoles are end diastolic. The P wave preceding the aberrant beat is not premature, but the ventricular complex is.

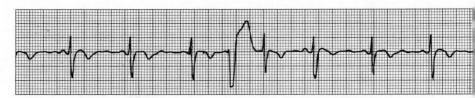

Fig. 10.   INTERPOLATED PVC. The basic sinus rate is 70. Therefore one would not expec
an interpolated PVC. Although delayed, the normal ventricular response i
not interrupted. There is also a wandering pacemaker. All the P waves are
not of the same shape. The flatter P waves are not premature but late. Thi
is the hallmark of the wandering pacemaker (a passive mechanism).

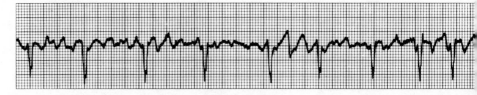

Fig. 11.   ATRIAL FIBRILLATION. There is a very coarse fibrillatory line, reflecting the lacl
of electrical unity in the fibrillating atria. If you thought that you saw I
waves, look for this same contour before each QRS and remember that P
waves of atrial flutter repeat their pattern throughout the tracing.

V₁

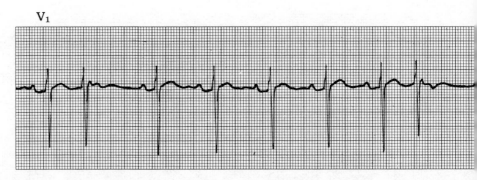

Fig. 12.   PREMATURE JUNCTIONAL COMPLEXES. There are two premature junctional beat
evident in this tracing. They are the second and the last complexes. Notice
that they are almost identical to the sinus-conducted beats and that they are
followed by a negative P′ wave, indicating that retrograde conduction to
the atria followed anterograde conduction to the ventricles.

II

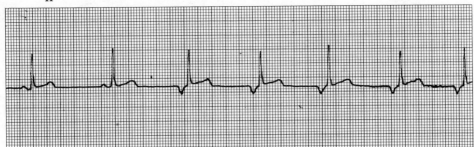

Fig. 13. SINUS BRADYCARDIA WITH A JUNCTIONAL ESCAPE RHYTHM. The underlying rhythm is sinus with a rate of 50. The escape junctional rhythm shows firing at a rate of 58. Note the change in polarity of the P wave when the pacemaker shifts from the sinus node to the AV junction.

V₁

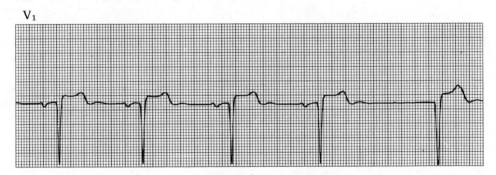

Fig. 14. SINUS BRADYCARDIA WITH SA BLOCK AND JUNCTIONAL ESCAPE. The junctional escape beat follows a long pause.

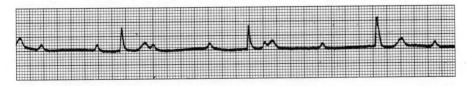

Fig. 15. COMPLETE HEART BLOCK. The P waves are clearly seen and occur regularly at a rate of 72. The ventricles are beating independently under the control of a nodal pacemaker at a rate of 32.

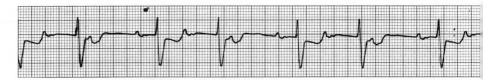

Fig. 16. SECOND-DEGREE AV BLOCK, TYPE I. The first P-R interval of each group is 0.28 sec. The second P-R interval is 0.48 sec, and the third P wave falls on the T wave and is not conducted. This is the cyclic prolongation of the P-R interval that describes second-degree AV block, type I (Wenckebach phenomenon). The QRS interval is also prolonged, indicating that there are lesions at two levels in the AV junction: at the AV node and at the bifurcation of the bundle of His.

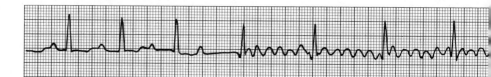

Fig. 17. SECOND-DEGREE AV BLOCK, TYPE I, FOLLOWED BY AN IDIOJUNCTIONAL RHYTHM AND ATRIAL FLUTTER. In the first part of the strip the P-R interval gradually increases from 0.20 to 0.36 sec, until finally there is nonconduction. The AV junction then begins to pace the ventricles at a rate of 57. Notice that the AV junctional complex is slightly different from the sinus-conducted beats. After the first junctional complex, one can see the typical sawtooth pattern of atrial flutter, in which the atrial rate varies from 325 to 400 beats/min. Because the AV junction is pacing the heart independently of the atrial ectopic rhythm, the ventricular complexes have no constant relationship to the flutter waves.

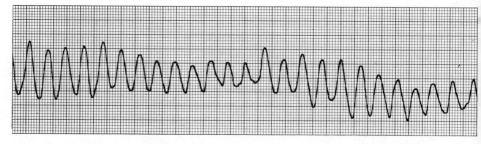

Fig. 18. VENTRICULAR FLUTTER. The ventricular rate is 225, and the complexes have become rounded and are no longer angular.

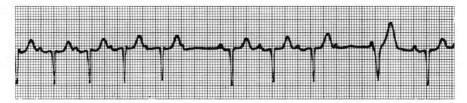

Fig. 19. SECOND-DEGREE HEART BLOCK TYPE I. A 4:3 Wenckebach sequence can easily be seen toward the end of this tracing. The P-R intervals lengthen until a P wave is not conducted. The P wave after this pause does not conduct either, since it is interrupted by a junctional escape beat.

Lead II

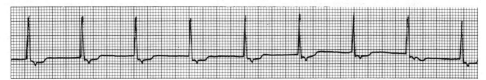

Fig. 20. AN ACCELERATED IDIOJUNCTIONAL RHYTHM. In lead II a negative P′ wave indicates a focus low in the atrium. If the P′ wave follows the QRS, the pacemaker is located in the AV junction and delayed retrograde conduction is present. This is not a normal escape mechanism, since the rate exceeds 60 beats/min. Such an accelerated junctional focus is commonly due to digitalis excess.

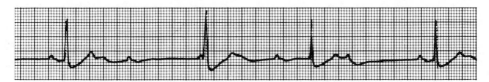

Fig. 21. SECOND-DEGREE HEART BLOCK (HIGH-GRADE) WITH JUCNTIONAL ESCAPE. At first glance this might appear to be a complete heart block. The ventricular rhythm, however, is irregular, and this should tell you to look for ventricular capture and junctional escape. The first and last complexes are conducted and have the same P-R interval. The second ventricular complex is an escape beat because the P wave is too close to conduct. The third R wave may or may not have been conducted.

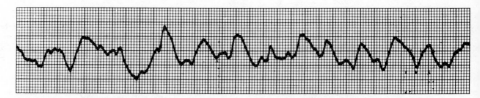

Fig. 22.   VENTRICULAR FIBRILLATION. Chaotic ventricular activity is reflected in this erratic ECG pattern.

Lead II

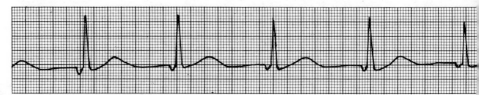

Fig. 23.   JUNCTIONAL ESCAPE RHYTHM. At a rate of 43 this is a passive escape rhythm. In lead II a negative P′ wave indicates retrograde conduction. The short P′-R interval (0.08 sec) indicates that the focus is below the AV node.

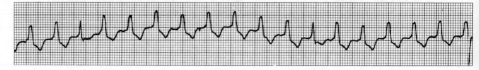

Fig. 24.   VENTRICULAR TACHYCARDIA. The rate of this tachycardia is 140. There are two Dressler (fusion) beats visible. These two factors are suggestive of a diagnosis of ventricular tachycardia.

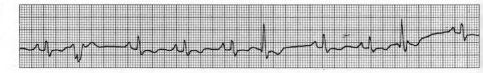

Fig. 25.   BIFOCAL PVCS. The basic rhythm is sinus conducted, and the rate is 75. The PVCs are of two different forms, indicating two foci in the ventricles.

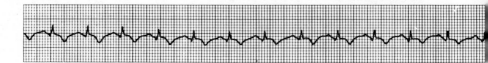

Fig. 26.   SINUS TACHYCARDIA. The rate is 122. Normal P waves are visible before each QRS complex.

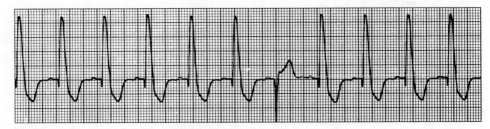

Fig. 27. VENTRICULAR FUSION. The P-R interval of the narrow complex is slightly less than the dominant P-R interval, indicating that an ectopic focus discharged in the ventricle just before the normal sinus stimulus reached the IV septum. The two vectors may meet, causing a complex of lesser amplitude and duration, or the ectopic focus may be of septal origin and may dominate the ventricles completely. The dominant rhythm is sinus tachycardia with BBB.

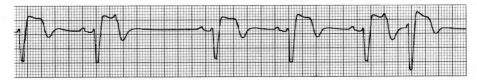

Fig. 28. PACS. There are two P′ waves in this tracing. Both occur during the S-T segment, and the first P′ wave is not conducted.

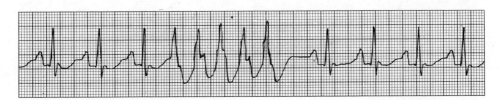

Fig. 29. PAROXYSMAL VENTRICULAR TACHYCARDIA. This burst of tachycardia begins with a PVC that remains in control of the ventricles for five beats. The sinus node then regains control.

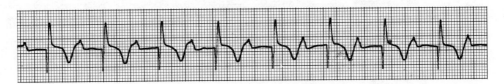

Fig. 30. FIRST-DEGREE HEART BLOCK. The P-R interval is 0.32 to 0.36 sec. All impulses are conducted but delayed across the AV junction.

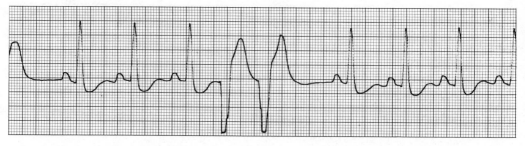

Fig. 31. PAIRED PVCS. This is a more ominous sign than the single PVC.

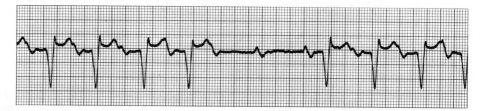

Fig. 32. SECOND-DEGREE HEART BLOCK, TYPE I. The nonconducted P waves furnish an opportunity to see the P-R interval of a conducted beat and the shape of the P wave. This is a second-degree A-V block because some of the P waves are not conducted. The P-R intervals lengthen until there are two dropped beats. The QRS interval is also prolonged (0.16 sec). The duration of the P wave is 0.16 sec, suggesting atrial hypertrophy.

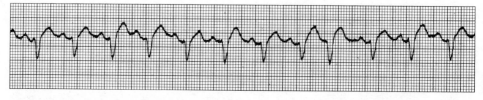

Fig. 33. SINUS TACHYCARDIA WITH PACS. The pause following the early ventricular complexes is not fully compensatory, indicating an atrial stimulus. The PAC causes the T wave in which it occurs to be taller and more peaked.

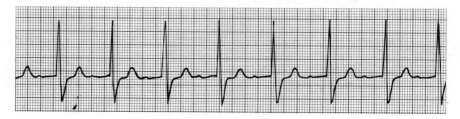

Fig. 34. FIRST-DEGREE AV HEART BLOCK. Both the P-R interval and the QRS interval are prolonged, indicating that the lesion involves the bundle branches.

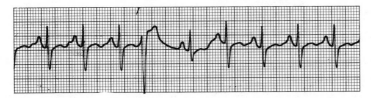

Fig. 35. SINUS TACHYCARDIA WITH A PVC. The sinus rate is 112.

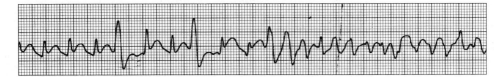

Fig. 36. FREQUENT PVCS RESULTING IN VENTRICULAR FIBRILLATION. At a rate of 160 the underlying rhythm is either a sinus or an atrial tachycardia. There are PVCs occurring very early in diastole. When they are finally paired, the result is ventricular fibrillation.

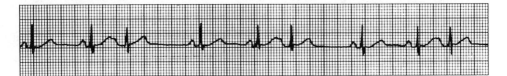

Fig. 37. TRIGEMINAL PACS. There is a PAC after each pair of normal sinus beats. The P′ wave distorts the preceding T wave. The P′-R interval is long (0.22 sec) because the ectopic stimulus occurs during the relative refractory period, causing a delay in conduction through the AV junction.

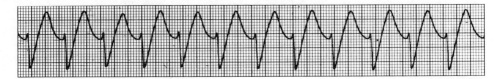

Fig. 38. VENTRICULAR TACHYCARDIA. The ventricular rate is 110. There are no P waves visible, and there are no ventricular fusion beats. This could therefore also be a supraventricular tachycardia with aberrant ventricular conduction.

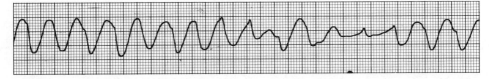

Fig. 39. VENTRICULAR FIBRILLATION. The onset of this tracing might be termed ventricular flutter, since there is some repetition of the wide, bizarre complexes. Complete electrical chaos soon is evident.

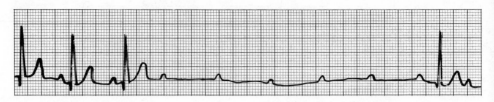

Fig. 40. SUDDEN COMPLETE HEART BLOCK WITH JUNCTIONAL ESCAPE. AV conduction abruptly fails in this tracing. The complexes at the beginning of the strip are conducted with a P-R interval of 0.16 sec. There is a long period with no ventricular activity and then junctional escape. This patient had Stokes-Adams syndrome and was a candidate for a pacemaker.

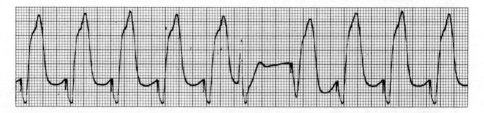

Fig. 41. DEMAND PACEMAKER. The pacemaker spike can be seen just before the ventricular complex. There is a PVC that is sensed by the pacemaker, and thus there is a delay in the next firing.

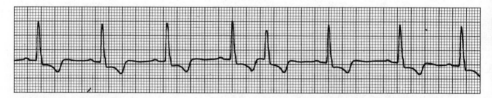

Fig. 42. PAC. The PAC in this tracing is not immediately apparent. The premature ventricular complex is not followed by a full compensatory pause. This causes one to search for a PAC. If the T waves are closely examined and their shapes compared, the inverted T wave preceding the premature complex appears to be more peaked. A P' wave occurs in the T wave.

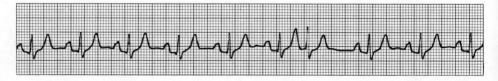

Fig. 43. PAC. The PAC in this tracing occurs on a T wave, causing it to be taller and more peaked.

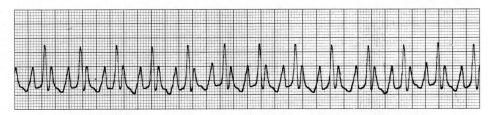

Fig. 44. ATRIAL TACHYCARDIA WITH 2:1 AV CONDUCTION. The atrial rate is 220. The ventricular rate is 110. One of the P' waves is partially hidden in the QRS complex. Its downstroke can be seen emerging from the S wave.

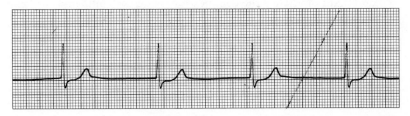

Fig. 45. JUNCTIONAL ESCAPE RHYTHM. The rate is 43. The P waves may be hidden in the QRS complex.

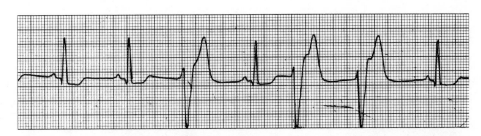

Fig. 46. FREQUENT, UNIFOCAL PVCs. The identical contour of these PVCs makes it evident that they are generated by the same ectopic focus. Additionally, because there is no exact coupling, you can suspect parasystole.

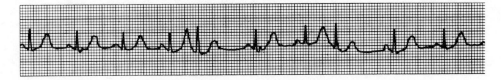

Fig. 47. PACs. The P' waves distort the preceding T wave and are both followed by normal ventricular conduction.

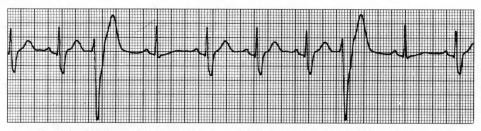

Fig. 48. PVCs IN ASSOCIATION WITH INTERMITTENT BUNDLE BRANCH BLOCK. The ventricular complex following the PVC is normal in contour and duration as opposed to the other sinus-conducted beats with their broad terminal S waves. This may indicate rate related BBB, since the PVC creates a longer cycle than the dominant one. Thus the complex following the compensatory pause is normally conducted.

Glossary

A

aberrant ventricular conduction A supraventricular impulse temporarily conducted abnormally within the ventricles, usually due to a change in cycle length and resulting in bundle branch block and/or hemiblock.

accelerated idiojunctional rhythm Enhanced automaticity of the AV junction at a rate greater than its inherent rate of 60 but less than 100/ beats min.

accelerated idioventricular rhythm Enhanced automaticity of the ventricular pacemaker cells at a rate greater than its inherent rate of 40 but less than 100 beats/min.

accelerated rhythm A rhythm (three or more consecutive impulses) of less than 100 beats/min but faster than the inherent rate of the ectopic pacemaker site, which is named. For example, accelerated junctional rhythm of 75 beats/min.

accessory pathway A muscular tract (one end inserts into conductive tissue) or connection (conductive tissue excluded) between the atrium and ventricle other than the bundle of His.

action potential Refers to the membrane potential and the changes it undergoes during the cardiac cycle.

   phase 0 The rapid depolarization phase of the action potential.

   phase 1 The early rapid repolarization phase of the action potential.

   phase 2 The plateau of the action potential.

   phase 3 The late rapid repolarization phase of the action potential.

   phase 4 The period between action potentials.

adrenergic Refers to the alpha and beta receptors for norepinephrine.

afterdepolarization A slow depolarization that follows a normal action potential and may itself elicit an action potential if it reaches threshold.

alert period (pacemaker) That time during which a pacemaker senses an R wave and emits a pulse if an R wave does not occur.

alpha and beta receptors The site on the muscle or gland where norepinephrine acts.

AN region Where the internodal tracts enter the AV node.

anions Negative ions.

antegrade conduction *See* **anterograde conduction.**

anterograde conduction Forward, that is, from atria to ventricles or from the AV junction to the ventricles.

arrhythmia Other than a normal sinus rhythm.

asynchronous pacing *See* **fixed-rate pacing.**

atrial synchronous pacing When pacing electrodes are both atrial and ventricular. The atrial electrode emits a pulse (in response to the P wave) that discharges the ventricular electrode.

atrioventricular (AV) dissociation When the atria and ventricles are under the control of independent pacemakers.

atrioventricular (AV) node Part of the conductive system of the heart in the posterior floor of the right atrium. It receives impulses from the atria and causes a delay before transmitting to the bundle of His.

automatic Spontaneous activity that arises without external cause.

automatic interval The interval between two consecutive pacemaker spikes during continuous ventricular pacing.

automaticity That property by which a cell can reach a threshold potential and generate an action potential without being stimulated from another source.

AV node *See* **atrioventricular node.**

axis (heart) The preponderant direction of current flow.

axis (lead) An imaginary line between the two electrodes of a bipolar lead or between the positive electrode and the reference point of the unipolar lead.

B

Bachmann's bundle Specialized conductive tissue from the anterior internodal tract into the left atrium.

beta receptors *See* **alpha and beta receptors.**

    beta$_1$ Refers to the beta receptors in the heart.

    beta$_2$ Refers to the beta receptors in the peripheral vasculature and the bronchioles.

bifascicular block Refers to right bundle branch block, with concurrent block in either the anterior or posterior fascicle of the left bundle branch.

bigeminy A series of two closely spaced complexes. The underlying mechanism should be specified.

bipolar electrode (pacemaker) A pacing electrode with a positive pole at its tip and a negative one behind that. Both poles are located in the heart (as opposed to the unipolar electrode).

blip A pacemaker spike.

block Failure or delay of conduction due to pathology.

bundle branch block (BBB) Delay or failure of conduction within a bundle branch. May be complete or incomplete, permanent or intermittent, or right or left.

bundle of His The conductive tissue connecting the AV node and the ventricles.

bypass tract A muscular connection between the atrium and ventricle that excludes the AV node.

C

capture Refers to a ventricular complex that has been conducted from a supraventricular source following a period of AV dissociation.

capture (pacemaker) Myocardium activated in response to an electronic pacemaker impulse.

catecholamines A specific group of vasoactive sympathetic endogenous mediators.

cations Positive ions.

chaotic rhythm *See* **multifocal rhythm.**

cholinesterase An enzyme responsible for the breakdown of acetylcholine.

chordae tendineae Strong, slender cords extending from the borders of the AV valves to the papillary muscles.

chronotropic Refers to heart rate.

competitive pacing *See* **fixed-rate pacing.**

concealed conduction Conduction within the AV junction, which does not result in a ventricular complex and is only detected because of its influence on subsequent impulse formation and/or conduction.

concealed WPW syndrome When conduction over an accessory pathway is possible only in a retrograde direction. *See also* **Wolff-Parkinson-White syndrome.**

conductivity The propagation of an impulse along a fiber.

connection A muscular pathway between atrium and ventricle excluding the conductive system (as opposed to a tract).

contractility The ability of cardiac fibers to shorten.

coupling interval The distance between two linked events in the cardiac cycle.

current of injury Occurs as a result of myocardial injury, resulting in elevation or depression of the S-T segment. May be either systolic or diastolic.

D

decremental conduction A gradual decrease in the stimuli and response along a pathway of conduction.

delta wave The initial slurring of the QRS complex found in Wolff-Parkinson-White syndrome.

demand interval The interval between two consecutive pacemaker spikes during consecutive spontaneous pacing.

demand pacing A pacemaker impulse is emitted only when the patient's R-R interval exceeds a preset limit.

depolarization Reduction of the resting potential of a cell to a less negative value. The process may be slow or rapid.

diastole (electrical) Phase 4 of the action potential.

diastole (mechanical) The relaxation of the heart.

diastolic current of injury The current that flows from injured to noninjured tissue during electrical diastole as a result of a reduction in membrane potential of the injured cells.

dromotropic Refers to AV conduction velocity.

dysrhythmia Other than a normal sinus rhythm. More correct than "arrhythmia" but less frequently used.

E

echo complex A complex resulting from a return of an impulse to its chamber of origin.

ectopic focus Other than the sinus node as pacemaker.

electrical alternans The alternating amplitude of QRS complexes commonly reflecting pericardial effusion.

electrogram *See* **His bundle electrogram.**

enhanced automaticity A speeding up of the process by which a pacemaker cell reaches threshold potential; a cause of arrhythmias.

entrance block Refers to delayed conduction or complete conduction block in the tissue surrounding a pacemaker site so that an impulse cannot enter and discharge that pacemaker. Such a pacemaker is said to be protected and may result in a parasystolic rhythm.

epicardial pacing Requires an incision so that the pacing electrode can be sewn into or screwed into the ventricle.

escape complex Discharge of a latent pacemaker because of undue delay in the dominant rhythm discharge.

escape interval The interval from the onset of a sensed QRS complex to the ensuing pacemaker spike.

escape rhythm Three or more consecutive impulses resulting from undue delay in the prevailing rhythm.

exact coupling Precise linkage of an ectopic complex to the preceding beat each time it occurs.

excitability (myocardial) The ability of a cell to reach threshold in response to a stimulus.

exit block Delay or failure of an impulse to activate the tissue surrounding the site of impulse formation.

external pacemaker A transvenous pacing catheter within the heart and attached to a pulse generator outside the body that is not implanted.

F

fibrillation-flutter Implies a supraventricular arrhythmia resembling both atrial fibrillation and atrial flutter. The term *atrial fibrillation* is preferred.

fixed-rate interval The interval between two consecutive pacemaker spikes after the application of a test magnet.

fixed-rate pacing Emission of a pacemaker impulse at regular intervals irrespective of the patient's own rhythm.

focal reentry Reentry resulting from dispersion of refractory periods.

fusion A collision of impulses within the atria or ventricles due to simultaneous activation of a chamber from two foci.

fusion complex (pacemaker) A collision of the supraventricular impulse with the pacemaker impulse within the ventricles.

H

H region The bundle of His excluding the tissue where the AV node converts to the bundle of His.

hexaxial figure When all lead axes on the frontal plane are drawn through the zero potential of the heart's electrical field.

high-grade, second-degree block Advanced second-degree block.

His bundle (bundle of His) The conductive tissue beginning at the lower part of the AV node and ending where the bundle branches begin, spanning the fibrous ring.

His bundle electrogram (HBE) A graph depicting the electrical events occurring in the AV node and bundle of His.

His-Purkinje system The conductive system from the bundle of His to the terminal ramifications of the interventricular conductive system.

hysteresis (pacemaker) When the interval following a sensed beat is different from (i.e., lags behind) the interval between paced beats.

I

inherent rate The normal rate of impulse formation at a given pacemaker site.

inotropic Refers to myocardial contractility.

interatrial tract *See* **Bachmann's bundle.**

internodal tracts Specialized conductive tissue connecting the AV node and sinus node.

interpolated complex When a PVC does not prevent conduction to the ventricles of the P wave immediately following it. There is not a full compensatory pause.

intranodal Within the AV node.

isorhythmic dissociation AV dissociation during which the atria and ventricles beat at approximately the same rate.

JKL

James bundle The posterior internodal tract at its distal end.

junction (AV) Composed of the AV node and the nonbranching portion of the bundle of His.

junctional tachycardia Enhanced automaticity of the AV junction resulting in rates over 100 beats/min.

Kent bundle Accessory pathways (connections) between atria and ventricles found on both sides of the heart.

Lown-Ganong-Levine syndrome A short P-R interval and normal QRS complex. The term *short P-R syndrome* is preferred by many.

M

macroreentry Reentry involving the bundle of His, both bundle branches, and the ventricular myocardium.

Mahaim fiber A fiber connecting the junctional region with the ventricular myocardium. A tract.

MCL$_1$ A bipolar chest lead that simulates the pattern seen in the unipolar lead V$_1$.

MCL$_6$ A bipolar chest lead that simulates the pattern seen in the unipolar lead V$_6$.

membrane responsiveness The relationship of the resting membrane potential at excitation to the maximum rate of depolarization.

microreentry Reentry within the Purkinje system of the ventricles.

Mobitz heart block, type I *See* **second-degree heart block, type I.**

Mobitz heart block, type II *See* **second-degree heart block, type II.**

Multifocal rhythm An atrial or ventricular rhythm emanating from more than one focus, as manifested by varying cycle lengths and complex morphologies.

NO

N region AV node itself excluding the tissue at its top, where the internodal tracts enter, and at its lower border, where the bundle of His begins.

NH region That portion of the conductive system where the AV node becomes the bundle of His.

nonpacemaker cell A cell without the property of automaticity.

nonparoxysmal tachycardia *See* **accelerated idiojunctional rhythm.**

oversensing (pacemaker) When the pacemaker senses P and T voltage, afterpotentials from the pacemaker pulse, and signals from outside the body.

overshoot When the action potential during phase 0 passes 0 mV and becomes positive.

PQ

P wave Represents atrial activation.

P prime (P′) A P wave that is generated from other than the sinus node.

pacemaker cell A cell exhibiting the property of automaticity.

parasympatholytic An agent that blocks the effects of the parasympathetic nervous system.

parasympathomimetic An agent that mimics the effects of stimuli to the parasympathetic nervous system.

parasystolic rhythm Refers to two sources of activation for one cardiac chamber, with one focus being protected from being discharged by the other because of entrance block.

paroxysmal atrial tachycardia (PAT) Refers to an AV nodal reentry mechanism. Paroxysmal supraventricular tachycardia is a preferred term.

paroxysmal supraventricular tachycardia An ectopic rhythm usually beginning with a PAC, PJC, or PVC and supported by an AV nodal reentry mechanism.

permanent pacemaker A transvenous or epicardial pacemaker with the pulse generator implanted in the subcutaneous tissue.

physiological refractoriness Refers to the normal period of inability to accept a stimulus; results in failure to conduct.

polarized cell The existence of ions of opposite polarity across the cell membrane.

potential (electrical) The energy possessed by a cell because of the ionic imbalance across its membrane.

P-R interval From the earliest onset of the P wave to the earliest onset of the Q or R wave.

preferential fibers Refers to intranodal fibers that conduct more rapidly than the normal AV nodal fibers.

preexcitation Activation of all or part of the ventricular muscle by an atrial impulse earlier than would occur if activation had proceeded normally through the AV node and bundle of His.

pumps (cellular) Refers to active transport of ions across the cell membrane.

Purkinje fibers Refers to the intraventricular conductive system excluding the bundle of His.

QRS complex Represents ventricular activation. Measured from the onset to the end of the widest complex.

QRS-inhibited pacemaker Refers to the pacemaker that does not fire at all when there are R-R intervals within a preset limit of time.

Q-T interval Represents repolarization of the ventricles. Measured from the onset of the Q or R wave to the end of the T wave.

R

recriprocal beat A ventricular or atrial complex that is the result of AV nodal reentry.

reciprocal changes Refers to the changes seen in leads facing the opposite wall to the myocardial infarction.

reciprocating The mechanism by which an impulse returns to the ventricle or to the atrium.

reentry Refers to the return of an impulse to or toward its origin.

refractory Unable to accept a stimulus.

refractory period
  effective That time during which excitation of a fiber is not possible; from phase 0 to approximately −50 or −60 mV in phase 3.

relative That time during which excitation and a propagated impulse is possible but only in response to a stronger stimulus.

repetitive firing Propagated action potentials that are the result of afterdepolarization.

repolarization Follows depolarization and consists in the return of the cellular potential to its resting value.

resting membrane potential The electrical charge across the cell membrane between impulses.

retrograde conduction Conduction in a reverse direction from normal.

ring pole The negative pole just behind the tip of the bipolar pacing electrode.

S

second-degree heart block A condition in which one or more P waves are not conducted to the ventricles; may be type I or type II.

second-degree heart block, type I (AV) When a nonconducted impulse is preceded by progressive prolongation of condition time. *See* **Wenckebach phenomenon.**

second-degree heart block, type II (AV) When a nonconducted impulse is against a background of constant conduction times.

sensing (pacemaker) The suppression of pacemaker output in response to electrical signals originating from natural ventricular activity.

short P-R syndrome When the P-R interval is less than 0.12 sec and the duration of the QRS duration is normal. Also known as Lown-Ganong-Levine syndrome.

sinoatrial (SA) node *See* **sinus node.**

sinus node Specialized tissue in the superior portion of the right atrium, the function of which is to pace the heart.

slow diastolic depolarization That property possessed by pacemaker cells which allows them to achieve threshold potential without outside stimulus.

slow inward current The slow depolarization of the cell, which is thought to be the result of a slow influx of calcium.

spontaneous activity Activity arising without external cause; activity that is intrinsic or automatic.

standby mode When the pacemaker is sensing normally and is inhibited by the patient's own beats.

standby (pacing) *See* **demand pacing.**

supernormal conduction Refers to conduction velocity that is faster than expected but not faster than normal.

supernormal period That interval in the cardiac cycle during which activation may result from a subthreshold stimulus.

supraventricular **(electrocardiographically)** Above the branching portion of the bundle of His.

supraventricular rhythm Any rhythm originating above the bifurcation of the bundle of His.

sympatholytic An agent that blocks the effects of the sympathetic nervous system.

sympathomimetic An agent that mimics the effects of stimuli to the sympathetic nervous system.

systole (electrical) From phase 0 to the end of phase 3 of the action potential.

systole (mechanical) Contraction.

systolic current of injury The current that flows from noninjured to injured tissue during electrical systole as a result of a shortening of the height and duration of the action potential of the injured cells.

T

T wave Represents ventricular repolarization.

tachycardia Three or more consecutive impulses at a rate exceeding 100 beats/min.

temporary pacemaker A transvenous pacemaker with the pulse generator not implanted.

third-degree heart block (AV) When all the conditions for AV conduction are present but conduction does not take place.

threshold (electrical) The smallest amount of electrical current needed to produce a propagated action potential.

threshold potential A critical value of intracellular negativity at which point the cell rapidly depolarizes to inscribe the upstroke of the action potential.

tip pole The positive pole at the tip of a bipolar pacing electrode.

tract A muscular pathway between atria and ventricle with one end inserted into conductive tissue (as opposed to connection).

transthoracic pacing Insertion of the pacing electrode into the ventricle with a transthoracic needle and a cannula.

trigeminy A series of three closely spaced complexes. The underlying mechanism should be specified.

triggered activity That repetitive activity of cardiac cells which is not due to inherent automaticity and is not in response to a stimulus outside itself. It is due to a slow depolarization following a normal action potential and termed an *afterdepolarization.*

UVW

U wave Follows the T wave. Possibly represents repolarization of the Purkinje fibers.

undersensing (pacemaker) Failure to sense a normal QRS complex.

unifascicular block When conduction does not occur in one of the three interventricular fascicles.

unipolar electrode (pacing) A pacing electrode with one pole at its tip within the heart and the other pole outside the body.

unipolarization The conversion of a bipolar pacing system to a unipolar one.

ventricular electrogram A recording of the QRS from an intracardiac site such as may be obtained with a pacemaker catheter.

ventricular standstill When the ventricles remain inactive.

vulnerable period That time during the T wave when some fibers are normal, some completely refractory, and others partially refractory, making reentry possible because of different conduction velocities within the ventricles.

Wenckebach phenomenon A prolongation of conduction time until conduction is finally blocked. Occurs in cycles.

Wolff-Parkinson-White (WPW) syndrome A short P-R interval, broad QRS complex, delta wave, and a tendency to paroxysmal supraventricular tachycardia.

type A When the delta wave is positive in V_1.

type B When the delta wave is negative in V_1.

Index

Boldface page numbers indicate the principal discussion of the subject.